the
complete
guide
to
NATURAL CURES

**Effective Holistic Treatments for Everything
from Allergies to Wrinkles**

DEBORA YOST

A Lynn Sonberg Book

HARPER

An Imprint of HarperCollins*Publishers*

This book contains advice and information relating to health care. It is not intended to replace medical advice and should be used to supplement rather than replace regular care by your doctor. It is recommended that you seek your physician's advice before embarking on any medical program or treatment. All efforts have been made to assure the accuracy of the information contained in this book as of the date of publication. The publisher and the author disclaim liability for any medical outcomes that may occur as a result of applying the methods suggested in this book.

HARPER

An Imprint of HarperCollins*Publishers*
10 East 53rd Street
New York, New York 10022-5299

Copyright © 2009 by Lynn Sonberg Book Associates
ISBN 978-0-06-145673-2

First Harper paperback printing: January 2009

Printed in the United States of America

Visit Harper paperbacks on the World Wide Web at www.harpercollins.com

10 9 8 7 6 5 4 3 2 1

TREAT YOUR MEDICAL CONDITION NATURALLY AND EFFECTIVELY

- **SKIN:** Acne, Age Spots, Athlete's Foot, Burns, Chapped Lips, Cold Sores, Eczema, Psoriasis, Sunburn, Warts, Wrinkles . . .

- **DIGESTIVE SYSTEM:** Belching, Constipation, Diarrhea, Flatulence, Gastritis, Heartburn, Irritable Bowel Syndrome, Ulcers . . .

- **HEART AND LUNGS:** Angina, Asthma, Bronchitis, Emphysema, Heart Disease . . .

- **EYE, EAR, MOUTH, NOSE, AND THROAT:** Cataracts, Earache, Glaucoma, Gum Disease, Laryngitis, Macular Degeneration, Sinusitis, Sore Throat, Toothache . . .

- **BONES, JOINTS, NERVES, AND MUSCLES:** Bursitis and Tendinitis, Carpal Tunnel Syndrome, Fibromyalgia, Osteoarthritis, Osteoporosis, Rheumatoid Arthritis . . .

- **AND:** Alzheimer's Disease, AD/HD, Cancer, Depression, Diabetes, Erectile Dysfunction, Fatigue, Gallstones, Headaches and Migraines, Hemorrhoids, Hypertension, Infertility, Insomnia, Parkinson's Disease, Prostate Problems, Stress, Varicose Veins . . . and *MUCH* more!

THE COMPLETE GUIDE TO NATURAL CURES

CONTENTS

the
complete
guide
to

NATURAL
CURES

1

TAKE CONTROL OF YOUR HEALTH THE NATURAL WAY

IF YOU ARE old enough to have medical issues, chances are you've noticed that health care isn't what it used to be.

In some ways, it is better. New advances in medicine are made every day. Less invasive ways are being found to diagnose disease better and earlier, which is saving lives and improving quality of life. The death rates from cancer and heart attack, among others, are dropping (though heart disease and cancer, respectively, are still the number-one and number-two killers).

Modern medicine in the United States is also embracing natural medicine like never before. Thousands of research studies are taking place at this very moment on the healing potential of herbs, plant foods, and other natural therapies. The federal government and some insurance companies are accepting the merit of alternative treatments and approving certain natural medicine techniques, such as chiropractic, acupuncture, and massage therapy. And it is becoming more common to find medical and natural physicians working in tandem to help patients.

In many other ways, though, health care is getting worse. Today, when you go to the doctor, your time is measured in minutes—*if* you are lucky enough to even be seen by a doctor, much less by *your* doctor. When you are truly in need of a doctor's care outside of office hours, your only recourse is to go to an emergency room and wait your turn.

Even the identity of your family doctor has become less of a sure thing. The "family doctor" you have this week may need to change to someone else next week because either your company has switched health insurers (which is happening an average of every two years) or your doctor has switched insurance carriers (which happens even more often). And it is not necessarily your doctor's fault—it is often the insurance company, not the doctor, making the decision. It's no wonder that "primary-care physician" has replaced the title "family doctor"!

How secure can you really feel that your doctor is acting in your best interest? You may have to go through unnecessary testing (though you'll never know it unless you ask) just so your doctor has a paper trail in case of a lawsuit, be it frivolous or one that has merit. The specialist you want to see (or your doctor would prefer you to see) and the "elective" surgery you need is often dictated by a third party—your insurance company—unless it is an emergency and your condition is life threatening. Even the medication you take is influenced by what your insurance company will allow and pay for.

Clearly, today's health-care system is far from ideal and if you're like most Americans you may no longer have easy access to a trusted family physician to answer all of your questions about common ailments and complaints. All the more reason to become informed about self-care and take control of your own health—which is what this book is all about.

HOW TO USE THIS BOOK

Many common health complaints can be managed effectively, safely, and efficiently on your own, using a variety of natural therapeutic approaches. In most cases, you can get significant relief from health problems as diverse as acne, back pain, bursitis, gout, and urinary tract infections without drugs and without going to the doctor. Using natural approaches not only puts you in control of your health, it also saves you time and money.

This book is designed to make you an informed health consumer and help you make decisions about your own health issues. However, it is not intended to make you a renegade. Rather, its message is this: While self-care is highly desirable, it may not always be your healthiest or safest route if certain symptoms arise or current symptoms get worse.

For example, you may use a certain herb to treat a sinus infection, but if your symptoms are getting worse instead of better, do not hesitate: call your doctor. Or, you may help relieve the symptoms of your emphysema with natural remedies, but this does *not* mean you should discontinue seeing your doctor or following your doctor's prescriptive advice.

This book is designed to be used by healthy adults. All dosages in this book are designed for adults and should not be given to children. If you are pregnant or nursing, you should not follow any of the advice in this book without the consent of your doctor. If you are taking any medication, prescription or over the counter, do not take any natural remedy without consulting with a qualified health-care professional. Certain medications and natural remedies can be dangerous when taken together. Also, do not stop taking a medication in favor of a natural remedy without consulting with your physician.

If you have a chronic or serious medical condition, discuss your natural healing options with your doctor. You should consider natural therapy only as a partner to your doctor's care. When you are under a doctor's care, it is your responsibility to keep him or her informed about your self-care. Your doctor cannot treat you properly if he or she is not aware of everything you are doing that affects your health.

Good self-care is based on being an informed natural-care consumer. To this end, every entry in this book gives you a basic understanding of the condition and how the recommended therapy works. Also, each section, where it is relevant, gives reasons and situations for which you should take your health care out of your own hands and put it in a doctor's hands.

All of the entries are organized alphabetically. You can use the table of contents or simply leaf through the book to find your "problem" and the natural therapies that should help. For instance, for "heartburn," you would look under *H* and for "constipation" you would look under *C*—the entries will not be found under "Digestive Ailments" or some larger category—each is listed individually.

The therapies suggested in this book focus on what is easy and practical to do on your own. They include nutritional supplements, herbs, homeopathy, and aromatherapy, plus sensible healthy-living practices. Before trying any of them, make sure you read the next chapter, which offers a basic understanding as to how these therapies are designed to work.

2

WHAT YOU NEED TO KNOW ABOUT BUYING AND USING NATURAL REMEDIES

THE ROOTS OF modern medicine are based in nature. Herbal medicine has been around as long as humans have inhabited the Earth. Traditional Chinese medicine has been practiced for more than four thousand years and embraces herbal and nutritional therapies. Ayurveda, the traditional Indian system of medicine, has been practiced since about 2500 B.C.

Naturopathy, which is based on the ancient belief that the body has the ability to heal itself, was developed in the late nineteenth century and brought to the United States from Europe in the late 1890s. In some ways it is similar to traditional Chinese medicine and to Ayurveda. In naturopathy, treatments focus on diet, herbs, hydrotherapy (the use of water to heal), yoga, and various physical therapies such as chiropractic, acupressure, massage, and reflexology.

In Europe, especially Germany and Great Britain, herbs for healing are dispensed as readily as pharmaceutical medications. In the United States, they are looked upon more as curiosities. Doctors in the U.S. are trained in allopathic, or conventional, medicine. They see a problem and seek to cure it or alleviate the symptoms with the latest and best pharmaceuticals. Alternative practitioners, on the other hand, seek to find the source of the problem, and prevent it from happening. Allopathic physicians depend on pharmaceuticals first to treat a health problem; alternative doctors depend on natural medicines, which are the source of many modern pharmaceuticals. But this is changing.

Today, allopathic doctors in the United States are paying attention to natural therapies like never before. As scientific studies on natural healing approaches prove that herbal and vitamin therapies have validity, conventional physicians are adopting some of the natural ways into their practices. And the public is embracing it. A recent survey by the National Center for Complementary and Alternative Medicine found that the majority of Americans have turned to some form of natural medicine to treat a medical problem.

Both allopathic and alternative medicine have a place in our lives. Herbs won't set a broken bone, so we must seek help from allopathic physicians, but herbs might speed healing and nutritional therapy might prevent it from happening again. Likewise, an allopathic doctor will help a patient with heart disease by monitoring heart rhythm, giving continual testing, and prescribing medications to lower blood pressure and cholesterol or to control heart rhythm. Natural physicians approach it with nutritional therapy, dietary changes, and stress-reduction techniques, such as progressive relaxation and yoga. Independently, neither is as effective as the two approaches used simultaneously.

There will be many circumstances in your life when self-care is appropriate. But in order to make an informed decision as to how to help yourself, you need to understand the type of therapy you intend to use. You must also respect its limitations. Know what you are doing before you proceed.

HERBAL MEDICINE

There is no doubt about it: herbal medicine can be effective medicine. But it is also strong medicine. People around the world have been using herbal remedies for thousands of years to treat ailments from the common cold to heart problems. Today, more than 80 percent of the world's population use herbs for health, although in the United States the figure is only around 20 percent.

The most important fact to keep in mind when it comes to natural remedies is this: Just because they are natural doesn't necessarily mean they are without risk. However, they are associated with fewer side effects than conventional medication. Problems with herbs generally arise if they are taken incorrectly, most notably in larger doses than are considered safe. They could also have a bad interaction with drugs you take. It is imperative that you know any and all risks before beginning alternative therapy.

When taking herbs as medicine, keep the following precautions in mind.

- If you are taking any medications, do not take an herb without consulting your doctor first. Certain medications and herbs do not mix.
- Do not stop taking a medication on your own in favor of taking a natural remedy.
- If you are pregnant or breastfeeding do not take anything—herbal or otherwise—without consulting with your doctor.
- More is never better. Stay within the recommended limit.

• The dosages for herbs (and other supplements) given in this book are intended for adults. Check with your child's doctor first before using an herbal remedy.

Side Effects and Reactions

Though reactions are rare if you follow instructions, some people can be allergic to certain herbs. If you know you have certain allergies, avoid herbs that are part of the family to which you have an allergy. For example, if you are allergic to bee stings, you do not want to take bee pollen.

Typical reactions, for the most part, are harmless. They include diarrhea, itching, or a rash. In the case of diarrhea, you should decrease the dosage or switch to something else. If you have a skin reaction, stop taking the herb and switch to an alternative.

Herb-Drug Interactions

Although herbs have been around centuries longer than most medications, experts know more about drug-to-drug interactions than they do about herb-drug interactions. Fortunately, research into herb-drug relationships is ongoing and new information is being released all the time. This is why it is imperative that you not mix herbs and medications without consulting an expert. Here, as an example, are a few known ways in which herbs can have an adverse effect when taken with common classes of medication.

Blood pressure medication. Certain herbs raise blood pressure and can do so even if you are taking medication to lower blood pressure. These include ephedra (ma huang), goldenseal, ginseng, licorice, hawthorn, and saw palmetto.

Antipsychotic medications. Herbs that treat depression or affect mood can increase the severity of psychotic symptoms and can also have a sedating effect. Herbs include St. John's wort, valerian, passionflower, and hops.

Corticosteroids. The herb licorice can increase the risks associated with taking the medication.

Nonsteroidal anti-inflammatory drugs. There is an increased risk of stomach bleeding when taking these drugs along with the herbs feverfew, garlic, and ginkgo biloba.

How to Buy Herbs

On occasion, you will find recommendations in this book for using fresh herbs or even those dried and prepared for culinary use. Most often, however, the herbal therapies called for are preparations that you can buy packaged in a health food store or pharmacy.

Packaged herbs come either processed or raw. Processed herbs include tablets, capsules, liquids (as tinctures and extracts), powders, teas, and creams. Raw, unprocessed remedies include dried roots, flowers, leaves, and stems. Many herbs come in more than one form. Use the kind recommended or the equivalent. When in doubt, ask someone knowledgeable about herbal medicine.

When buying herbs, follow these guidelines.

- Look for herbs labeled *organic*. This assures that no pesticides or herbicides were used during harvesting or preparation.
- Check the label to see what part of the plant was used, for example, the roots or the leaves. If a remedy in this book identifies a specific part of the plant, make sure that this is what you are buying.
- The label must provide specific dosages and directions for taking the herb.
- Before you buy, read the label. Check for an expiration

date and a lot number. The use instructions should be clear. Read the dosage instructions.

• Make sure the herbs are packaged with a safety seal and that the seal is not broken.

• Look for the words *standardized extract*. This means that the potency of the active healing component of the herb is guaranteed.

How to Store Herbs

For starters, store medicinal herbs as you would pharmaceutical drugs: out of the reach of children. Also, follow these guidelines.

• Store all herbs in a cool, dry environment and out of sunlight.

• Keep loose, dried herbs in an airtight container.

• Keep capsules and tablets in their original containers and make sure to keep lids tightly closed.

NUTRITIONAL THERAPY

Since you care enough about your health to be reading this book, you already know that good nutrition is the foundation of good health. For the body to function properly, it must have a sufficient supply of more than forty key nutrients. While few Americans suffer from severe deficiency diseases such as scurvy or rickets, the Council for Responsible Nutrition reports that most Americans do not consume adequate amounts of many nutrients, including vitamins A, B6, B12, C, D, E, thiamin, riboflavin, and folic acid, and the nutrients calcium, chromium, iron, magnesium, selenium, and zinc. These inadequate intakes may not trigger a disease directly caused by a nutrient deficiency, but they leave the body vulnerable to an array of other diseases and chronic conditions, including many of the diseases and ailments you will find in this book.

Food is not only fuel for the body, however. It is medicine as well. Scientific research has revealed a lot about nutritional supplements over the last few decades. While the body is dependent on essential vitamins and minerals to sustain life, newer studies are proving that these and other nutrients are just as important in enhancing health and fighting off disease. They include certain amino acids, enzymes and hormones; essential fatty acids; a long list of antioxidant phytonutrients; and other natural compounds you will read about in this book.

Why You Need Supplements

Unfortunately, the typical American diet is deficient in nutrients and fiber and high in fat, cholesterol, and preservatives. Even if you include lots of fresh fruits, vegetables, and whole grains in your diet, you may not be consuming as many nutrients as you think. Most nonorganic foods grow in nutritionally deficient soil, which generates nutritionally deficient produce. Furthermore, between the time the food leaves the field and reaches your dinner plate, additional nutrients are destroyed by food processing, storing, and cooking.

To make matters worse, your body may not be able to take advantage of all the nutrients you do consume. Emotional and physical stress can cause a breakdown of your immune system and make you susceptible to invasion by harmful microorganisms and result in countless problems, from the common cold to ulcers to heart disease, all of which can hinder how your body absorbs or uses nutrients. Stress also increases your body's requirements for many nutrients, especially the water-soluble vitamins such as vitamin C and the B vitamins. That's why, for example, you can buy vitamin combinations sold as "stress formulas," which contain the B vitamins and often vitamin C as well.

In addition, the process of aging increases the body's demands for nutrients. As you age, your body loses some of its ability to assimilate the nutrients you consume. For example, research shows that as you get older, levels of important nutrients start to decline. These include certain amino acids, such as methionine and cysteine; the antioxidants coenzyme Q10 and vitamin E; and certain hormones, such as DHEA (dehydroepiandrosterone). Ironically, your body's demand for these nutrients increases at the same time your physical reserves drop. Supplementation is one solution. Though nutritional supplements cannot stop the aging process, more and more studies show that taking certain supplements can stall the aches and pains and diseases that generally go along with getting older.

Of course, what you eat does matter . . . and all the supplements in the world will not make up for a poor diet.

Whenever possible, you should make an effort to obtain a given nutrient from actual food as well as from the recommended supplements.

Please see Appendix A, *Food as Medicine* (page 247) for a handy summary of the best food sources of various nutrients.

Knowing Your Nutrients

Nutritional therapy is not a matter of simply increasing your intake of certain vitamins and minerals. Other nutrients, such as amino acids, enzymes, natural hormones, phytonutrients, essential fatty acids, and food itself are instrumental to healing and play a key role in this book. Here is a brief summary of these nutrients and the roles they play in your health.

Vitamins and Minerals

Vitamins and minerals are essential to life. Without vitamins and minerals, the body would not be able to function.

Each has a key role in maintaining one or several roles in keeping organs and every single cell in the body functioning. Unlike other substances (such as hormones), the body does not manufacture its own vitamins and minerals and must depend on food to get an adequate supply. This is why the federal government, through the Federal Drug Administration (FDA), has identified the amount of each essential vitamin and mineral that is necessary to sustain life. While many still refer to it as the RDA (Recommended Daily Allowance), it is now referenced on labels as the DV (Daily Value).

Keep in mind, however, that the DV is the amount that is required to sustain life and avoid a nutritional deficiency. It is also based on what one dosage contributes nutritionally to a hypothetical 2,000-calorie-a-day diet. Optimal levels to enhance health and avoid disease are generally higher. This is why you will find that the recommendations in this book do not coincide with the DV. They are, however, considered safe for the average, healthy adult. For example, the Daily Value for vitamin C is 60 milligrams for men and women (on a hypothetical 2,000-calorie-a-day diet). Optimal levels are considered anywhere from 500 to 1,500 milligrams a day.

Vitamins are also divided into two main groups: fat soluble and water soluble. Fat soluble means that a certain amount of body fat is required to absorb and store the nutrient. Because these nutrients are stored in fat, they remain in the body for use as needed. This is no storage space in the body for water-soluble vitamins, meaning the body takes what is needed and excretes what's left.

The fat-soluble vitamins are A, D, E, and K. Vitamin A can be toxic at high levels, which is why nutritional experts recommend beta-carotene, a precursor to vitamin A, as nutritional therapy. Beta-carotene is not harmful in high dosages. The water-soluble vitamins include vitamins B and C.

Use the DV as a point of reference when taking vitamins or minerals as nutritional therapy. These are the DVs for the vitamins and minerals recommended in this book. They are for men and women only. DVs are smaller for children and greater for pregnant and lactating women.

Nutrient	Men	Women
Vitamin A	1,000 R.E.	800 R.E.
Vitamin C	60 mg	60 mg
Vitamin D	200 I.U.	200 I.U.
Vitamin E	10 mg	8 mg
Biotin	30 mcg	30 mcg
Folate	400 mcg	400 mcg
Niacin	16 mg	14 mg
B6	1.3 mg	1.3 mg
B12	2.4 mcg	2.4 mcg
Calcium	1,000 mg	1,000 mg
Copper	1.5–3 mg	1.5–3 mg
Iron	10 mg	15 mg
Magnesium	420 mg	320 mg
Selenium	70 mcg	70 mcg
Zinc	15 mg	12 mg

Phytonutrients

Phytonutrients are naturally occurring substances found only in plant foods. They are not essential to life, but in the last few decades scientists have discovered they may be more powerful than vitamins and minerals when it comes to enhancing health and fighting disease. Many medicinal phytonutrients are found in the skin of the plant and can be identified by their rich colors. Carotenoids, for example, are found in yellow-orange fruits and vegetables, such as carrots and sweet potatoes.

Phytonutrients, also called phytochemicals, mostly work as potent antioxidants and powerful detoxifiers. Scientists have discovered that certain phytonutrients not only exceed the antioxidant properties of vitamins, but can even enhance their healing powers.

Hundreds of phytonutrients have been discovered in the last two decades, and scientists believe there could be thousands more yet undiscovered. Certain classes of phytonutrients have distinct healing abilities. The ones you'll find in this book include the following.

- Carotenoids
- Lignans
- Isoflavonoids, flavanols, and flavones
- Phytoestrogens
- Indoles
- Limonoids
- Polyphenols and phenolic acids
- Lycopene

Amino Acids

Amino acids are the building blocks of protein and, like vitamins and minerals, they are essential to life.

Amino acids play a key role in your daily health. Almost every structure of the body requires continuous resupply of amino acids to maintain healthy tissue and organs.

The body depends on around 20 amino acids and manufactures all but nine on its own. These nine are referred to as the essential amino acids because they must be obtained from foods that contain protein.

Amino-acid therapy is an emerging field of nutritional

science because scientists believe that the body's need for amino acids increases with exposure to disease, toxins, and stress.

The amino acids recommended as supplements in this book include the following.

- Arginine
- Gamma-aminobutyric acid (GABA)
- Glutamine
- Lysine
- Taurine
- Tyrosine

What Labels Tell You

In 1994 legislation was passed requiring manufacturers to provide key information about the contents of their products on all packaged food and supplement products. You can find this on the back of the supplement box and container as the *Supplement Facts* label.

The federal government, however, is not a watchdog over supplement companies like it is over drug companies. But this does not mean there are no controls. Look for the acronym *USP* on the label, which means the product meets standard labeling requirements of the United States Pharmacopeia.

The USP is an independent nonprofit organization that was established in 1820 to determine the quality, purity, packaging, potency, and labeling standards for drugs and nutritional supplements. It is comprised of representatives of more than 100 various medical institutions, national associations, and federal government departments. A product that has *USP* on its packaging means it meets the standards of the organization.

However, there is no federal regulation that governs the

potency or purity of vitamins and herbs you buy. You should buy your supplements from a company that you trust.

HOMEOPATHY

Homeopathy is based on the German-born concept that "like cures like." Basically the concept says that a substance that causes symptoms of an illness or disease in a healthy person can also be used to treat the same symptoms in a sick person.

The principle is similar to the one used by mainstream medicine when it comes to vaccinations. To prevent the measles, or polio, for example, you inject someone with a tiny amount of measles or polio virus. Similarly, in homeopathy, a remedy contains a minute amount of the substance that, in much higher dosages, would cause the illness.

Like other natural therapies, homeopathy works with the healing mechanisms within the body. Homeopathic medicines are prescribed not just for the disease itself, but also for the symptoms that are expressed with a certain disease.

Homeopathic remedies are prescribed in two ways: A single remedy prescribed by a trained homeopathic physician, or as a combination formula that is prepared and packaged for common conditions and sold in health-food stores. These combination formulas have been found to be safe and effective and are the only homeopathic remedies recommended in this book.

If you're interested in homeopathy, you would do best to go to a homeopathic physician for treatment advice and guidance. There are, however, some basic homeopathic formulas that have been proven safe for self-treatment. You can find them most places nutritional supplements are sold. The homeopathic recommendations in this book are limited to these proven products.

Caring for Homeopathic Medicines

When taking homeopathic medicines, follow these guidelines.

- Take at least 15 minutes before or after eating.
- Substances such as toothpaste, chewing gum, tobacco, and mouthwash can counteract the effect of the remedy. Some practitioners advise against caffeine while taking a remedy.
- Take with a clean, dry spoon, or a dropper.
- Do not chew tablets or granules. Let them dissolve in your mouth.
- Store remedies in a dark, cool place.

AROMATHERAPY

Aromatherapy involves the use of essential oils, which are concentrated from the roots, stems, leaves, seeds, and flowers of medicinal plants. They have been used as healing agents since 4500 B.C.

Aromatherapy is based on the principle that when essences are inhaled or applied to the skin, they connect with chemical messengers and travel to the ailing site or organ. Numerous studies support the effectiveness of essential oils in enhancing the immune system and fighting bacteria, viruses, fungi, and other microbes that invade the body.

Essential oils are very concentrated and, therefore, very potent. Only tiny amounts are needed to get the healing effect. Some are also dangerous; they are not to be taken by mouth. They can also be harsh and cause a skin reaction.

Essential oils are not oily, as their name suggests. They are actually rather fragile and evaporate quickly, leaving no residue.

For all these reasons, essential oils that come in contact with the skin are generally mixed with carrier oils. These carriers can be any type of oil—olive, almond, and sunflower are common—or basic unscented lotion.

Using Essential Oils

The rule of thumb for an aromatic bath is 30 drops of essential oil to 7 tablespoons of carrier oil. For massage oil, mix 8 to 12 drops of essential oil to 6 to 8 teaspoons of carrier oil.

For respiratory conditions, essential oils are generally used full strength, either by putting a drop or two on a tissue and inhaling or inhaling directly from the bottle. To steam with essential oils, put a few drops in a bowl of hot water, place a towel over your head, and inhale the vapors.

Because essential oils are fragile substances, you should buy them in small amounts. Buy and keep them in a dark glass vial. Look for the words *pure* or *true* on the label, which indicates that the oil was derived from an organic plant. Store your essences in a cool, dark place and uncap the oils only long enough to release the amount of oil you need to keep the oil from evaporating.

BE PREPARED

Many of the conditions in this book are for common illnesses or incidents that come on suddenly or overnight, like motion sickness or a cold. When you are feeling lousy is not the time to go to the store in search of self-healing agents. Be smart and keep some basics around the house so they are there when you need them. These include the following.

- Ginger
- Garlic
- Unscented lotion
- Aloe vera—preferably the plant
- Chamomile essential oil or tea

- Echinacea tincture, tablets, or tea
- Black tea
- Lavender essential oil
- Honey
- Lemon
- Olive oil
- Vitamin E capsules
- Vitamin C

An A to Z Guide
to Natural Cures
for Common Ailments

ACNE

There are pimples . . . and then there is *acne*.

Though we think of acne as a teenage rite of passage, it can rear its ugly blackheads, whiteheads, and pustules at any age. And, ironically, it seems to attack those who fear it most—women.

Acne targets women for the same reason it is the scourge of adolescents, especially teenage boys: hormones. In youths, of course, the underlying cause is raging testosterone levels and in girls it is estrogen. Women can experience a breakout as a result of the hormonal fluctuations that accompany menstruation, pregnancy, and especially menopause. Yes, acne can follow you clear through middle age!

So, why are some people plagued with acne-prone skin while others can sail through life with nothing more than an occasional pimple or two? The reason, experts say, is heredity.

COMMON CAUSES

There are a lot of old wives' tales as to what triggers an acne attack—most notably chocolate and greasy foods—but evidence indicates that food sensitivity is purely a personal thing. There is evidence, however, that points to a nonfood suspect: stress.

When you're under stress, your body releases high levels of hormones to help you handle the situation at hand. One such hormone is cortisol, which triggers the pancreas to pump glucose into the bloodstream. Although scientists aren't sure why stress causes acne, one theory holds that cortisol aggravates the sebaceous glands under the skin, which, in turn, produces excess sebum, an oily substance designed to lubricate the skin.

Another possible cause of acne is overzealous use and lackadaisical removal of foundation and concealing makeup. Doctors even have a name for it—*acne cosmetica*. Even water soluble products can get trapped in pores and clog your skin's "breathing room," which only exacerbates problems for acne-prone skin.

BLEMISHES DEFINED

Blemishes result when sebaceous glands run amok and cause an overproduction of sebum. Too much sebum can clog the pores, which show up on the skin as blackheads. When bacteria grow beneath the skin, the glands release enzymes that break down the sebum. The result is whiteheads. You don't have true acne, however, until these blemishes become inflamed and cause pustules that can ooze and even be painful.

Most of the skin's sebaceous glands—and most cases of acne—are located on the face, back, chest, and shoulders.

Acne wouldn't be considered problematic if it could disappear overnight. But there are plenty of things you can do on your own to smooth out the bumpy road to a clear complexion. Just be patient and give these remedies time to work. It may take up to three months to see permanent results.

SMOOTHING SOLUTIONS

Tea tree. The oil from the tea tree plant acts as a natural antiseptic and has been found to be as effective against acne as over-the-counter benzoyl peroxide but without the irritation and drying effects. Just put a few drops of tea tree essential oil on a cotton pad and dab it on your trouble spots three times a day. Or, make a tea tree acne lotion by combining three parts essential oil to one part nonoily, nonfragrant lotion.

You can cut corners by looking for a commercial lotion containing tea tree, but it most likely won't be as effective as using the concentrated essential oil.

Chasteberry. Herbalists have been using chasteberry, also known as vitex, to regulate hormones—both male and female—for centuries. According to herbal lore, monks in the Middle Ages regularly drank chasteberry tea to keep their libidos under control. It is still commonly used to help control the side effects of premenstrual syndrome.

If your skin erupts in unsightly bumps when you are having your period or you notice acnelike changes in your skin during menopause, try sipping a cup or two of chasteberry tea a day. But don't overdo it; herbalists say that more than two cups a day might make the condition worse. Relaxing with a cup of tea is also a nice way to destress.

SUPPLEMENTAL HELP

Zinc. Studies have found a correlation between acne and low levels of zinc. The mineral has several beneficial functions associated with acne. It helps regulate hormones, promotes wound healing, and is essential to vitamin A metabolism. It also helps regulate insulin.

At one time, zinc was administered for acne in therapeutic doses, which must be done under medical supervision. However, some doctors report notable improvement with 30 milligrams, three times a day. This is considered in the safe range—the daily value is 15 milligrams and high-potency vitamins can contain up to three times that amount. But check with your doctor first, as too much zinc can be toxic.

Vitamin A. The well-known acne prescription drug Accutane is a derivative of vitamin A, which is essential to healthy skin. Studies show that high doses of vitamin A can be just as effective as Accutane. Vitamin A, however, is fat soluble, meaning it can build up in your system and become toxic. It is better to stick with a multivitamin containing 4,000–5,000 I.U. of vitamin A, and make sure you eat plenty of foods containing vitamin A, such as carrots, sweet potatoes, broccoli, and winter squash.

Chromium. This trace mineral helps metabolize sugar, meaning it might help your acne if excess blood sugar is contributing to the problem. Check to make sure your multivitamin contains 200 micrograms of chromium.

Vitamin E. There is anecdotal evidence that vitamin E, which is found in vegetable oils and nuts, is beneficial for mild cases of acne.

Recommended dosage: 400 I.U. a day.

The vitamin team. Many vitamins work better synergistically; zinc and vitamins A and C are on this list. If you have any kind of skin problem, make sure your daily multivitamin contains adequate but safe dosages of these nutrients. Also, eat foods high in these nutrients.

Flax. Flaxseed—as food, oil, or supplement—has numerous health advantages, and one of them is healthy skin. Flax is an excellent source of omega-3 fatty acid, which can help guard against acne in two ways: it helps prevent sebaceous glands from overproducing sebum and it also helps reduce skin inflammation.

PAY ATTENTION TO PREVENTION

Consider what you eat. While there is debate as to whether greasy and sugary foods cause acne, there is evidence that certain foods can cause a pimple or two to pop in susceptible people. If you suspect a certain food is aggravating your skin, eliminate it from your diet for several days, then reintroduce it and see what happens.

Go natural. *Must* you wear makeup all the time? At least a few days a week, face the day with nothing more than a good cleansing (no soap!) and a thin coating of moisturizing cream containing sunscreen.

Water down your makeup. Toss any oil-based makeup, which is hard to remove, in place of water-based makeup.

Don't ever, ever skip your facial routine. Whatever you do, don't go to bed without removing your makeup and cleansing your skin. Your skin needs breathing room, and cells replenish themselves while you are asleep.

Water your skin. Drink plenty of water every day to help keep your skin from drying out. Better yet, drink it with a squeeze of fresh lemon. Citrus is good for the skin.

WHEN TO CALL THE DOCTOR

If natural remedies don't offer any improvement after three months, consider seeing a natural physician who specializes in vitamin therapy. Or, see a dermatologist for a complete evaluation.

If you have oozing and painful sores that don't get better with natural solutions, see your primary-care physician or dermatologist. You may require antibiotics.

AGE SPOTS

Freckles tend to be cute. Some even consider them a sign of beauty. But age spots? Cute they're not.

Age spots are manufactured the same way freckles are: the skin produces excess pigment that appears a tone or two darker, especially after a good dose of sunlight. Rather than appearing as cute little dots, however, age spots show up as large, brown splotches, usually on the face and hands.

Despite their name, age spots aren't a result of old age;

they are a result of sun damage. As with age-promoting wrinkles, it takes decades for them to show up.

Certain drugs can accentuate or bring on age spots prematurely. These include the antibiotic tetracycline, blood pressure medication, diuretics, and drugs to control diabetes.

There is no need to wear the error of your ways like a scarlet letter. You may not be able to erase the past, but you can help make it fade.

AGE ERASERS

Aloe. The gel of the aloe vera plant has been proven effective against radiation burns. It promotes healing by sloughing away damaged skin and encouraging the growth of new, healthy cells. By extension, it may have the same effect on age spots. Just break off the tip of one of the plant's spines and apply it directly to the spots once a day.

Buttermilk. The lactic acid in buttermilk can have a similar effect. Coat a cotton ball with buttermilk and swab it on age spots morning and night.

Yogurt and honey. Together they make natural bleach. Blend one part plain yogurt and one part honey and rub it on with your fingertips. Let it dry thoroughly, then remove. Repeat daily.

Vitamin E. You can help reduce future damage by neutralizing age-making free radicals that are released from the sun with vitamin E oil. Break open a capsule and apply it *after* sun exposure.

PAY ATTENTION TO PREVENTION

Screen the sun. It's never too late to practice prevention. Stay off the beach or golf course from 10 AM to 2 PM when the sun is the most damaging and always, always apply a sunscreen any time you're going to be in the sun. Make wearing a sunscreen a daily habit, especially if you live in the Sunbelt.

WHEN TO CALL THE DOCTOR

Age spots are harmless and do not require medical attention. However, if the spots get irritated, sore, or change in an adverse way, it is wise to get them checked out by a dermatologist. What appear to be age spots to the untrained eye could be initial signs of skin cancer.

ALLERGIES

An allergic reaction happens when your immune system acts like firefighters responding to a false alarm as if it were a ten-alarm blaze.

With an allergy, the false alarm is a harmless substance that your immune system perceives as a threat to the safety of your health. Inside your body a team of reactors known as immunoglobulin E (IgE) antibodies try to thwart the threat with a flood of substances known as histamines. This sets off a chain reaction that leads to any of a number of uncomfortable symptoms.

ALLERGIES MOST COMMON

Allergies come in an almost infinite variety, but most fit into one of three categories: airborne, contact, and food allergies.

The most common are airborne allergies, which produce symptoms such as sneezing, nasal congestion, coughing, itchy throat, and watery eyes. The biggest offenders are dust, pollen, pet dander, and mold. Pollen allergy is commonly called hay fever.

Contact allergies cause skin irritation, which can show up as a rash, itching, or other skin eruptions. Common offenders include wool, fabric softener, perfume, and nickel found in inexpensive costume jewelry.

Food allergies, or sensitivities, are among the toughest to

solve, as symptoms are not always immediate. The range of foods someone can be allergic to is wide, but common allergens include dairy foods and wheat or gluten. Some food allergies, such as peanuts and shellfish, can be life threatening.

Finding the source of an allergy often takes quite a bit of detective work, especially when it causes obscure symptoms, such as headache, fatigue, and water retention.

Common pharmacological intervention includes decongestants to open up nasal passages and antihistamines to suppress the body's release of symptom-causing histamine. Most, however, have uncomfortable side effects, most notably sleepiness and lethargy. You can get the same benefits, without the side effects, by taking herbs or other supplements and practicing smart prevention tactics.

RELIEF FOR AIRBORNE ALLERGIES

Stinging nettle. Preparations made with freeze-dried nettle leaves are one of the best-known and effective natural remedies for hay fever symptoms.

Recommended dosage: Take 500 milligrams of freeze-dried leaves in capsule form three times a day during hay fever season.

Garlic. This member of the allium family contains several compounds with anti-inflammatory properties. Garlic is a great source of quercitin, a bioflavonoid that helps open nasal passages. Eat ample portions of fresh garlic in food. Or you can take garlic tablets.

Recommended dosage: One capsule twice a day while symptoms last.

Onions. Another quercitin-containing member of the allium family. If you love onions, take advantage of eating them during hay fever season.

Quercitin. If hay fever hits you hard, considering taking quercitin straight in capsule form.

Recommended dosage: Take 200 to 500 milligrams a day while symptoms last.

Wasabi. There is nothing like a shot of this potent Japanese horseradish to clear the sinuses. If wasabi is too much for you to handle, go for prepared horseradish. An easy and tasty way to take it is atop an oyster cracker.

Eyebright. You can drink it or use it as an eye solution to soothe sensitive peepers.

Recommended dosage: Dilute 5 drops of tincture with an ounce of saline solution and apply a drop or two with an eyedropper three times a day.

CONTACT ALLERGIES

Chamomile. You can soothe itchy skin and irritation with a lotion containing chamomile essential oil. Make sure to buy German chamomile.

Other essential oils. Lemon and peppermint essential oils also can help relieve itchy skin. Look for lotions containing these oils.

Flaxseed oil and fish oil. People with problem skin due to allergies may benefit from taking one of these oils.

ALL ALLERGIES

Vitamin C. This popular vitamin has natural antihistamine powers. A review of more than 25 vitamin C studies found that people who regularly take vitamin C supplements have fewer allergy complaints.

Recommended dosage: Take 1,000 milligrams of vitamin C with bioflavonoids throughout the day.

PAY ATTENTION TO PREVENTION

The best way to deal with allergies is to avoid exposure to the substances that trigger outbreaks. To keep the air around you clean, consider these ideas.

- Keep your home dust free—and vacuum with an appliance that uses a HEPA air filter.
- Use vinegar and water as a natural antiseptic to wipe down counters and cabinets.
- Change filters on your air conditioners regularly.
- Keep windows closed and the air conditioner on (if needed) during hay fever season.
- Keep plants away from doors and open windows to prevent pollen from getting into the house.
- Decorate your home with clean-air plants, such as dracaena, peace lily, and spider plant.
- Bathe your pets regularly and keep them out of the bedroom.
- Cover your box spring, mattress, and pillow with covers designed to repel allergens.
- If you have a damp basement, run a dehumidifier at all times.

WHEN TO CALL THE DOCTOR

Anaphylactic shock is a severe life-threatening allergic reaction that is most commonly associated with bee stings but it can occur in response to other allergens as well.

The appearance of hives (welts), wheezing, and trouble breathing are possible signs of a medical emergency. Do not delay—seek medical help right away.

ALZHEIMER'S DISEASE

It is one thing to forget your house keys but it's quite another to forget that you even have a house.

Such lapses in the order of everyday living are often the early signs of Alzheimer's disease, the gradual deterioration of the brain that results in a continuous decline in mental and even physical functions.

Alzheimer's disease, which afflicts more than four million Americans (including two out of three nursing home patients), not only robs a lifetime of memories, but also cruelly takes away quality of life—not just for those afflicted with the disease, but for their caregivers as well.

CROSSED WIRING

Alzheimer's occurs when the nerve fibers around the hippocampus, the brain's memory center, become crossed and knotted, making it impossible for the brain to store or retrieve information. In addition to this internal short circuit, the brain also experiences a drop in important neurotransmitters, including acetylcholine, which further breaks down the body's communication network. Researchers have found that people with Alzheimer's also have an acetylcholine deficiency.

Unfortunately, experts do not fully understand the cause of Alzheimer's disease, although there does appear to be a hereditary link. They do know, however, that autopsies on the brains of Alzheimer's patients show higher than normal levels of aluminum, calcium, silicon, and sulfur.

Some researchers speculate that the blood protein apolipoprotein E (apoE) may play a role in the disease. The presence of this protein is determined by genetics, and one of its forms, apoE4, has been associated with a higher risk of Alzheimer's. It is unclear whether apoE4 destroys the nerve cells in the brain or if it is involved with plaque formation.

So far there is no cure for Alzheimer's and no known way to reverse or stop progression of the disease. All therapies, both conventional and natural, aim to slow the advancement of the disease and ease symptoms. Some of them specifically target acetylcholine.

ACETYLCHOLINE TARGETS

Rosemary. This memory-enhancing herb contains compounds that prevent the breakdown of acetylcholine. Drinking rosemary tea may have some benefit in helping slow memory loss in those with Alzheimer's.

Lecithin. Lecithin contains choline, the precursor to acetylcholine. You can get a daily dose of lecithin by eating Brazil nuts, soybeans, fava beans, lentils, fenugreek greens, and poppy seeds.

MEMORY MAKERS

Ginkgo. One study involving 40 patients with early signs of Alzheimer's disease found that ingesting 240 milligrams of ginkgo biloba extract daily helped slow decline in memory. Ginkgo helps by increasing blood flow and oxygen supply to the brain. The active ingredients responsible for this action are flavonoid compounds known as heterosides. Allow four to six weeks to see results.

Recommended dosage: 60–80 milligrams of gingko three times daily.

Carnitine. Italian studies have found that this amino acid, in the form of L-acetyl-carnitine, can slow the rate of mental decline in people with Alzheimer's disease.

Recommended dosage: 500 milligrams three times daily of L-acetyl-carnitine.

Phosphatidylserine. PS is an important brain nutrient that helps balance brain chemistry and cell-to-cell communication and has been shown to improve memory when taken in therapeutic dosages. It may also be helpful in battling Alzheimer's disease. Most people get 50–80 milligrams a day from food sources, such as soy foods, rice, and fish. Studies show that dosages up to 300 milligrams a day are needed to guard against Alzheimer's disease.

Recommended dosage: Up to 300 milligrams of PS a day.

Vitamin E. This antioxidant helps prevent free radical damage to brain cells. Taken early enough, it may help prevent Alzheimer's or slow its progression. One study followed 341 people with Alzheimer's disease who were given a prescription drug, 2,000 I.U. of vitamin E, or a placebo for two years. The researchers found that people taking vitamin E were 53 percent less likely to reach the advanced stages of Alzheimer's disease than those in the placebo group. The vitamin E group fared better than the prescription drug group, too.

Recommended dosage: Take 400 I.U. daily as a preventative and 800 I.U. daily if early signs of Alzheimer's disease are already present.

DHEA. This natural hormone, which declines with age, is known to improve memory and mental abilities when taken in doses up to 50 milligrams daily.

PAY ATTENTION TO PREVENTION

Alzheimer's disease, and other diseases associated with progressive loss of mental acuity, such as senile dementia, is not a normal or inevitable part of aging. In generally healthy people, intellectual performance can remain relatively uncompromised well into the 90s, provided the mind remains active and stimulated. As a rule, older people do not lose a significant amount of their mental ability, and if they do, it is usually a result of a physical problem, such as a stroke.

WHEN TO CALL THE DOCTOR

If you or a loved one experience persistent forgetfulness, short-term memory loss, disorientation, and loss of train of thought, bring it to the attention of your doctor. Though it may indicate early signs of Alzheimer's disease, it mostly likely is age-related dementia.

Dementia, or senile dementia, refers to general mental deterioration including memory loss, moodiness, irritability, personality changes, childish behavior, difficulty communicating, and inability to concentrate. Alzheimer's disease is a severe type of dementia.

ANAL FISSURES

Some of the medical "firsts" in life are hard to forget. Like your first black eye, your first broken arm, your first trip to the operating room, or your first anal fissure. In fact, when you have an anal fissure, you are reminded of it every day, especially when you try to make a bowel movement.

Anal fissures aren't serious, but they are troublesomely painful. Some say it is like trying to pass a double-edged knife.

A fissure results when the lining of the anus tears when you are trying to pass an unusually hard or large stool.

Anal fissures are most common among young people who have poor diets, a stressful schedule, don't take the time to yield to nature's call and end up constipated. When the time does come, their less-than-elastic anal canal can't take the pressure, and it rips, making future trips to the bathroom hard to handle.

Unfortunately, anal fissures are slow to heal, but there are a few solutions to ease the pain—and prevent fissures from returning.

TENDER TREATMENTS

Psyllium. Psyllium is still considered Mother Nature's state-of-the-art solution for constipation and hard stools. It is found in over-the-counter powders such as Citrucel and Metamucil. Check the label before buying to make sure the product contains psyllium and take according to package directions.

Vegetables, fruits, and grains. These natural foods all contain fiber, which most likely is what is lacking in your diet and the origin of your problem in the first place.

Recommended dosage: Nine servings of fruits and vegetables and at least a cup of whole grains a day.

Goldenseal. Soothe anal fissures with a balm made out of this herbal antibiotic. Mix one tablespoon of the powdered herb with just enough olive oil to make a sticky paste. Apply it to the outside of the anus and the inner tears.

Aloe. Use aloe gel the same as you would goldenseal balm.

Water. Drink plenty of water—at least 8 full glasses a day. Water is essential as a bulking agent to produce soft stools.

WHEN TO CALL THE DOCTOR

Anal fissures can cause tears that bleed. This in itself is not a medical concern. However, blood on bathroom tissue should always be a concern, as it can be a sign of cancer. If in doubt, call your doctor.

ANEMIA

Has your "get up and go" got up and gone? If so, chances are you could have iron-deficiency anemia, or what doctors used to call iron-poor blood.

Iron is a mineral essential to the production of hemoglobin, which transports oxygen through the blood. Without enough hemoglobin, cells don't get enough oxygen, which causes the brain, muscles, and other tissue to slow down. Iron also is involved in the enzymatic action that produces human energy. When your iron stores are low, you end up feeling weak and dragged out, without enough energy to get you through the day. You may feel headachy and have trouble concentrating.

Iron deficiency is most common among women, who require more iron than men due to blood loss during menstruation and the body's increased iron needs during pregnancy. Other common causes are poor diet, excessive dieting, fad diets, and lifestyles that restrict or eliminate animal products. Vegetarians are at risk because the most accessible type of iron, heme iron, is found only in animal foods.

There are other forms of anemia, but iron-deficiency anemia is the most common. It is something you can also remedy on your own. You cannot, however, diagnose it on your own. You will need to see your doctor for a blood test, which is the only way to recognize for sure that you have an iron deficiency.

FOOD THERAPY

If bad food choices are to blame for your anemic condition, then better food choices can help you correct the problem. Follow these iron-rich practices.

Beef up. Meat is the best source of available heme iron, and calf's liver contains the highest iron content. Though liver was expelled decades ago as a good-for-you food due to its high fat and cholesterol content, your doctor most likely will give you a special dispensation, at least for the short term. Calf's liver can be quite tasty when properly prepared, so take advantage of this special treat. Just don't add any extra fat, especially butter, in its preparation.

Sauté in cast-iron pans. You'll get an iron bonus when you cook food in cast-iron pans. Foods cooked in cast iron actually absorb some of the minerals from the pan, which is then passed on to you. Studies have found that you can nearly double your absorption of hard-to-absorb non-heme iron (found in plant sources) when you consume vitamin C foods at the same meal.

Eat oranges with your meat. Or any citrus fruit that is high in vitamin C. Vitamin C enhances the absorption of iron.

Pass on the spinach salad. Spinach is a great source of calcium. Problem is, calcium also interferes with the body's ability to absorb iron. The solution? Do not eat calcium-rich and iron-rich foods at the same meal.

Avoid foods containing oxalic acid. This substance, found in foods such as almonds, asparagus, beans, beets, cashews, chocolate, kale, and rhubarb, also interferes with iron uptake.

Be careful of what you drink. The tannins found in black tea and coffee interfere with iron absorption.

A SUPPLEMENT PLAN

Iron. If you're iron deficient, your health-care provider will most likely have you take iron supplements. Make sure to buy iron marked as citrate, fumarate, glycinate, or succinate, as these are the most absorbable forms.

Recommended dosage: The typical recommendation is 30 milligrams two to three times a day.

Vitamin C. As noted above, vitamin C enhances iron absorption. Take up to 500 milligrams a day with your iron tablet.

Spirulina. The United States is the largest producer of blue-green algae, but U.S. residents, ironically, are not commonly known to use spirulina. This member of the seaweed family assists in the production of red blood cells. It is sold in supplement form.

Recommended dosage: Up to 2,000 milligrams a day.

Stinging Nettle. The leaves of this herb are rich in iron. Take it as a tea. Mix 1 teaspoon of powdered herb per cup of boiling water. Steep for 10 to 20 minutes and strain. Drink no more than one cup daily.

Ashwagandha. Also known as Indian ginseng, Ayurvedic physicians have been using it for thousands of years. It is believed to have numerous healing powers, including the ability to help purge anemia by increasing the production of hemoglobin.

Recommended dosage: Up to 2,000 milligrams a day.

WHEN TO CALL THE DOCTOR

If you suspect you are anemic, do not start an iron-supplement program without first getting a blood test from a qualified health-care practitioner. This is the only way to diagnose iron deficiency. You will also need to get additional blood tests because excess iron can be toxic.

Iron deficiency is not only the most common form of anemia, it is also the most benign. Other types of anemia, such as pernicious anemia, hemolytic anemia, sickle cell anemia, and thalassemia, are serious blood disorders that need to be treated under medical supervision.

You should also be under a physician's care for anemia if you also have heart disease or any other condition that involves the blood.

ANGINA

Do you feel like a thousand-pound gorilla is sitting on your chest? Chances are you have angina, a crushing, tightening chest pain that is telling you that your heart isn't getting enough oxygen-rich blood.

Many people who get angina for the first time think they are having a heart attack. The only difference—*usually*—is that the constricting pain of angina will ease when you stop what you're doing.

Angina means that your arteries are not squeaky clean and a buildup of plaque is causing blood to slow down on its way to the heart when you exert it too much. Most angina attacks occur when the heart is stressed by physical exertion, emotional upset, excessive excitement, or even digesting a heavy meal. Walking outside on a cold day, running to catch a train, or hearing particularly distressing news can bring on attacks. Angina attacks serve as painful reminders that the heart has been damaged, and a full-blown heart attack may follow unless steps are taken to mend your ailing heart.

If you've already been diagnosed with angina, your doctor probably has advised you to carry little nitroglycerin tablets, which you should take when you feel an attack coming on. *These pills are important.* Here is what you can do in addition to taking your nitro and to help make these episodes fewer and farther between.

HELP-YOUR-HEART SUPPLEMENTS

Coenzyme Q10 (CoQ10). Some 75 percent of people with angina also have a deficiency of this substance, which is present in every cell in the body and aids in the production of energy. In one study people who took CoQ10 cut the frequency of their attacks in half.

Recommended dosage: 150 milligrams twice a day.

L-carnitine. This amino acid helps the heart use oxygen more efficiently. Studies show that people who take carnitine supplements can significantly improve their ability to exercise without getting an angina attack.

Recommended dosage: 500 to 1,000 milligrams three times a day.

HELP-YOUR-HEART HERBS

Hawthorn. Sometimes referred to as a "heart tonic," this is the herb most often prescribed to help ease angina. Widely used in Europe, it works by dilating the coronary arteries and improving blood circulation in the heart.

Take a commercially prepared product or take it as a tea using 2 teaspoons of crushed leaves per cup of boiling water. Steep 20 to 30 minutes, strain, and drink up to two cups per day. Hawthorne is considered a powerful heart medicinal, so check with your doctor before taking it.

Willow. Willow bark is herbal aspirin, and aspirin has been shown to help prevent heart attacks. A cup or two of willow tea daily is the equivalent of low-dose aspirin. Take it only with the okay from your doctor.

Kudzu. In one of several Chinese studies, people who took 10 to 15 grams of kudzu root extract a day for 4 to 22 weeks showed a reduction in angina attacks. Kudzu is known to dilate arteries, increase blood flow, and stabilize heart rhythm.

COMMON SENSE SOLUTIONS

Stop! Cease whatever you are doing when an attack comes on. If you are racing around, slow down. If you are walking, sit down. If you are lying down, change your body position.

Stay calm. Close your eyes and breathe slowly but deeply. Concentrate on something pleasant and serene.

Get out of the cold. Cold weather can sometimes trigger an attack. Get yourself in a warm place or position as soon as possible.

Don't exert yourself. Sudden exertion, even lifting a heavy object, can bring on an attack. Approach everything as you should life in general: slowly and thoughtfully.

PAY ATTENTION TO PREVENTION

The only way to avoid angina is to keep the heart and circulatory system healthy. A healthy heart requires a healthy body.

- If necessary, lose weight.
- If you smoke, stop.
- Exercise regularly—that is, a minimum of three times a week.
- Eat a well balanced diet containing plenty of antioxidant-rich deep green and orange vegetables.
- Eat fish rich in omega-3 fatty acids three times a week.

WHEN TO CALL THE DOCTOR

First-time angina should not be self-diagnosed. If you feel tightness or pain in your chest, or pain radiating into your arm or back, *even if it goes away quickly,* report it to your doctor right away.

Angina is a symptom of heart disease, not a disease in its own right. If you experience chest pain, make an appointment with a cardiologist for a complete physical.

ANXIETY

Anxiety isn't all in your head. It visibly exists all over your body. Trembling limbs, a racing heart, sweaty palms, clammy skin, dry mouth, shallow breathing, incessant babbling, and even a flood of tears are all signs of apprehension, panic, and fear that express themselves as anxiety.

We all feel anxious now and then, but uncontrolled anxiety or panic attacks can be debilitating and terrifying experiences, lasting from a few minutes to several hours or days.

In some cases, the episodes become chronic and ongoing, interfering with the ability to live a happy and productive life.

Along with the physical symptoms, a person experiencing an anxiety attack typically feels an overwhelming sense of terror or impending doom.

Unlike fear in response to danger, anxiety is an expression of a generalized, undefined fear. The physical and emotional symptoms can be so severe and terrifying that people who experience anxiety attacks often end up in the hospital emergency room, convinced they are having a heart attack.

While there is considerable debate about the causes of anxiety attacks, many experts suspect that a neurochemical imbalance can trigger both anxiety disorders and depression. (People who are prone to depression also tend to experience anxiety attacks.)

Anti-anxiety medications are among the most prescribed drugs in America but they also have a long list of nasty side effects. Chief among them is dependency. Before considering the pharmacological solution, try one of the many natural remedies that have stood the test of time in helping to soothe nerves and banish irrational fears.

HERBAL CALM

Valerian. Researchers suggest that certain compounds found in valerian root bind to the same brain receptors as the anti-anxiety drug Valium, hence its nickname "natural Valium."

Valerian has a somewhat nasty taste, so it is best to take it in capsule form. It not only will calm your nerves but it also will make you sleep better.

Recommended dosage: 150 milligrams twice a day.

Kava. This herb contains several compounds believed to have a positive effect on the brain and nervous system. One study found that it increases secretion of gamma-amino-butyric acid, also known as GABA, which promotes relaxation. Herbalists recommend taking it in capsule form; as a tea it can cause stomach upset.

Recommended dosage: Up to 500 milligrams for anxiety.

Chamomile. Though not as effective as kava or valerian, chamomile is probably the most popular herb used to soothe raw nerves. One reason is its pleasant taste.

It is most popular as a tea. For best results (and the best potency), brew it fresh. Steep a teaspoon of dried chamomile flowers in a cup of boiling water and let it steep. One cup will go a long way to calm you down. Drink one cup of tea three times a day.

Tip: Fresh chamomile doesn't maintain its freshness very long, so buy it in small quantities.

Better yet, add several drops of chamomile essential oil into a tub of warm water. Dim the lights and take a relaxing bath.

Passionflower. This climbing vine grows wild in the South. It contains flavonoids, which have anxiety-releasing qualities. Unlike other herbs, it doesn't have a sedating effect, so it is a practical herb to take when you want to be calm but also need to be alert and mentally at your best.

Recommended dosage: 500 milligrams in capsule form twice a day. You can also drink it as a tea. Steep 1 teaspoon of dried passionflowers in 8 ounces of brewed water and steep whenever you're feeling anxious.

St. John's Wort. This well-known herb, which is widely used to treat depression, can also help those who suffer from anxiety.

Recommended dosage: Take 300 milligrams as an extract three times a day to soothe nerves.

Magnesium. This mineral has a tranquilizing effect.

Recommended dosage: 500 milligrams a day as needed.

PAY ATTENTION TO PREVENTION

You may not be able to eliminate anxiety from your life, but you can help minimize its frequency and intensity by making these techniques a habit.

Take a deep breath. In fact, take several deep breaths. Belly breathing goes a long way in helping reduce anxiety. This is how to belly breathe: Put your hand on your stomach and slowly inhale. Feel your belly expand. Hold your breath for a few seconds and slowly exhale.

Exercise. Aerobic exercise is a well-known anxiety reliever. When you're all tense and worried and don't know what to do, get your body in motion: Go for a jog or take a long, brisk walk—anything that takes your mind somewhere else.

Meditate. Studies show that transcendental meditation is the proven path to tranquility. If you're a nervous Nelly, consider finding a teacher or a class to learn this age-old practice.

Avoid alcohol. Resist the urge to reach for a drink during anxiety-building moments. In the end, alcohol can have the opposite effect.

WHEN TO CALL THE DOCTOR

Prolonged, severe anxiety can have serious consequences for your health. If anxiety attacks are so frequent that they are taking a toll on your daily life, talk to your doctor or seek the help of a professional counselor.

Anxiety can also have potentially serious underlying causes, such as hyperthyroid disease or a tumor.

ASTHMA

Breathing is something most people take for granted. The exception is the 17 million Americans who have asthma.

For reasons not completely understood, people with asthma have hypersensitive airways that constrict or get blocked when they sense environmental irritants that don't bother normal lungs. Mild attacks cause wheezing, shortness of breath, a buildup of excess mucus, and difficult breathing. Severe asthma attacks can be downright frightening because it feels like you can't breathe at all. They land nearly half a million people in hospitalization each year.

Each case of asthma is unique. Triggers can vary from person to person. Common triggers include smoke, dry air, cold, and common allergens such as mold and pollen.

If you have asthma, you most likely carry with you an inhaler (bronchodilator), a device that can offer immediate relief in the event of a sudden attack. You may even take medication to control attacks. You should continue these practices.

It is not well understood why certain people develop asthma or why asthma has become more common over the past two decades, especially among children. What is better understood are measures that can control and help prevent attacks. Asthma doesn't have to put major limits on your life. There are many things that you can do to take control of your asthma and minimize its impact on your activities.

AIR FRESHENERS

Fish. Studies show that children who eat fish containing omega-3 fatty acids more than once a week have a third of the risk of getting asthma than children who do not eat fish. Fish oil helps suppress the inflammation involved in the disease. If you don't get enough fish in your diet, take fish oil capsules.

Recommended dosage: 5,000 to 10,000 milligrams a day.

Flaxseed. Flaxseed oil is an alternative way to get a daily dose of essential fatty acids.

Recommended dosage: One or two tablespoons a day.

Onions. Onions contain substances called thiosulfinates that help inhibit inflammation associated with asthma. Avoid pickled onions, however, as they contain sulfites, a common trigger for asthma attacks.

Quercitin. This bioflavonoid is a natural antihistamine and is included in allergy relief combination formulas. It helps suppress the same irritants that trigger allergies. Onions, by the way, are a good food source of quercitin.

Recommended dosage: 400 milligrams 5 to 20 minutes before each meal.

Vitamin C. Studies have found that people with asthma tend to have low levels of vitamin C in their blood. Studies also have found that people with asthma who routinely take vitamin C tablets have fewer attacks. One study found vitamin C helps cut attacks by nearly 75 percent.

Recommended dosage: 1,000 milligrams of vitamin C daily.

Astragalus. This powerful immune booster helps suppress respiratory problems. It also helps strengthen the lungs.

Recommended dosage: 500 to 1,000 milligrams twice a day.

Vitamin B6. People with asthma tend to have low levels of this essential nutrient. One reason is that some asthma medications can reduce vitamin B6 levels in the body. One study found that taking B6 supplements dramatically decreased frequency of attacks and severity of symptoms.

Recommended dosage: 25 to 50 milligrams twice daily.

Ginkgo. One study found that ginkgo biloba extract, which contains anti-inflammatory and antioxidant agents, decreased the severity of asthma symptoms.

Recommended dosage: Take 150 to 200 milligrams a day.

Oregano. This popular pizza flavoring is used by homeopathic physicians to reduce the symptoms of asthma. Try getting more of it in your diet.

PAY ATTENTION TO PREVENTION

The first and most important order of wellness is to remove all the triggers in your daily environment that can lead to an asthma attack or cause symptoms. To this end, you should keep an account of your attacks and what you were doing at the time in order to help identify new or suspected triggers. Other practical techinques include the following.

- Avoid sudden exposure to cold air. When going outside in the winter, protect your respiratory system by wrapping a scarf around your neck.
- Avoid powerful odors, such as perfumes and strongly scented foods.
- Don't smoke and avoid second-hand smoke.
- Keep a distance from fireplaces and wood-burning stoves.

WHEN TO CALL THE DOCTOR

Call your doctor if attacks begin to get more frequent and you need to use your inhaler more often.

If you get a severe attack in which you are gasping for breath, get to the emergency room immediately.

ATHLETE'S FOOT

Athlete's foot is an equal opportunity afflicter. It can brand its signature itching, cracking, burning, and soreness on the feet and between the toes of couch potatoes as well as jocks.

This is because athlete's foot is a highly contagious fungal infection that thrives in any warm, moist environment, such as showers, restrooms, locker rooms, and inside of sneakers, socks, and ordinary shoes. It can even show up on sandals with synthetic insteps if you wear them too long on a hot day and get sweaty feet. In fact, sandals can make you more vulnerable because bare feet put you that much closer in contact with the fungus.

Using a contaminated towel or stepping infected feet into underwear can cause the infection to show up in another warm environment. When this happens it is called jock itch.

If you've recently been on antibiotics, you may be more susceptible to picking up this fungal infection because the drugs, in addition to fighting the cause of the infection, also kill the good bacteria that help resist fungus.

You can short-circuit an attack of athlete's foot with these natural remedies.

FIERCE FUNGUS FIGHTERS

Licorice. This herb reportedly contains more antifungal compounds than any other plant. Steep three or four tablespoons of the dried herb in several quarts of water and bring it to a boil. Let the brew warm and pour it into a shallow pail for a footbath. Soak your feet for 20 minutes once or twice a day until the symptoms are gone.

Garlic. Fresh garlic also contains abundant fungal-fighting compounds (though not as many as licorice). Take a footbath by pressing several cloves into warm water and soak your feet for 20 minutes. Be forewarned, however, as it may leave a lingering odor.

You can also steep crushed garlic in olive oil and dab it between your toes and on your feet with a cotton ball.

Tea tree. The oil from this herb is a well-known remedy

for athlete's foot. Mix equal parts of tea tree oil and vegetable oil and apply it on sore toes and feet with a cotton ball several times a day.

Goldenseal. This herb contains two alkaloids that have antifungal properties. Add a half ounce of powdered goldenseal to two cups of boiling water. Steep for 15 minutes. Let the mixture cool to a warm temperature and add it to a shallow basin for a footbath.

BE DIET WISE

Avoid sugar and yeast. Fungus breeds on these two substances so eliminate them from your diet.

Go probiotic. Replace friendly bacteria by eating it. Probiotics are good bacteria found in lactobacillus acidophilus and lactobacillus bifidus. The live cultures are found in yogurt.

PAY ATTENTION TO PREVENTION

If you are susceptible to athlete's foot, take strides to keep your feet as clean and dry as possible. Wear white cotton socks that allow feet to breathe, and wash the socks in chlorine bleach after each wearing to kill any fungus that might be present. Also, don't wear the same pair of shoes two days in a row. Shoes absorb moisture and need time to dry out.

If you tend to have sweaty feet, change your socks several times daily, and whenever possible, wear sandals or open-toe shoes to allow air to reach your feet. And, of course, wear waterproof slippers or sandals in locker rooms and public showers to avoid contact with the fungus.

WHEN TO CALL THE DOCTOR

Athlete's foot can usually be defeated by consistent and aggressive home treatment. The fungal infection can be accompanied by a bacterial infection, however, which might require medical attention. If the condition persists or gets worse after one month of treatment, call your doctor.

ATTENTION DEFICIT/ HYPERACTIVITY DISORDER

Statistics show that the rate of emotional and behavioral problems among young children is escalating at alarming rates. More than 20 percent of today's children go to school each day on some kind of prescription psychiatric drug. And, according to government statistics, there is another 20 percent that isn't receiving any medical treatment at all.

The majority of these children are on the drug Ritalin, the most commonly prescribed psychiatric drug for attention deficit/hyperactivity disorder (AD/HD), the most common mood-related childhood disorder. The use of this stimulant drug has increased a staggering 800 percent since the 1990s, and it appears that there is no end in sight.

Yet, Ritalin is not without controversy. Its critics say the drug is overprescribed, has undesired side effects, and can lead to addiction. Its proponents say that its benefits far outweigh its risks. Yet, there is one fact that can't be challenged: its long-term effects are still unknown.

WHO HAS AD/HD?

AD/HD is loosely defined as exhibiting actions and behavior inappropriate to developmental age. This includes the inability to focus, lack of concentration, learning disabilities, acting out, aggressive behavior, and poor social skills.

Unfortunately for parents, however, there is no medical test—mental, physical, or otherwise—that diagnoses AD/HD. A diagnosis is purely subjective and usually based on the number of behavioral-symptom displays and the degree of learning deficit.

Also unknown are the causes of AD/HD and the reasons for the rising incidence. But there is growing evidence that the cause is environmental and everything from poor diet to pollutants to the decline of the traditional family structure has been indicted. Childhood infections, traumatic birth, and genetics may also play a role.

There is also evidence that prescription drugs are not the sole solution. Parents have experienced success with some of these natural strategies.

A DIETARY BALANCE

Put the whole family on a whole foods diet. Studies show that poor diet probably has the most negative impact on a child's behavior. Substances such as additives, preservatives, and processed sugars and grains are like foreign invaders to the digestive system and blood of the human body, which was designed to run most efficiently and effectively on Mother Nature's food. Refined sugar is notorious for contributing to hyperactive behavior in children. One overlooked culprit is the sugar load in natural fruit juices that well- intentioned mothers give their children in place of soft drinks.

Look for food sensitivities. Many children with AD/HD have sensitive or underdeveloped digestion systems. This means that your hyperactive child could be allergic to any number of foods, even natural foods. This is not the type of allergy that causes an immediate reaction, as found with such foods as peanuts and wheat. Food sensitivities can cause behavioral reactions that can take hours or even days to manifest. You can try to pinpoint food sensitivity by removing a suspected food from your child's diet for several weeks, then reintroducing it. Monitor your child's behavior and mood for changes over the next several days.

Check your child's vitamin and mineral status. Children with AD/HD are often fussy eaters. Deficiencies in an essential vitamin or mineral can affect behavior. Protect your child's nutritional status with a high-potency multivitamin appropriate for your child's weight and age. In addition, make sure your daily menu contains foods that supply the following nutrients.

- *B vitamins, calcium, and magnesium.* These nutrients help relax the nervous system.
- *Vitamin C.* This antioxidant can help release toxins in the body that might be contributing to your child's behavior.
- *Iron.* Iron deficiency has been linked to the inability to concentrate.
- *Zinc and copper.* Deficiencies of both nutrients have been linked to ADHD.
- *Essential fatty acids.* It may be hard to get your kids to eat fish, but give it a try. Essential fatty acids found in fish are good for the brain.

NUTRITIONAL SUPPLEMENTS

Phosphatidylserine. Commonly called PS, this natural substance is important to brain health and is recommended by natural doctors as an alternative to Ritalin.

Recommended dosage: 200–300 milligrams a day.

GABA. Gamma-aminobutyric acid is an amino acid that has a calming effect on the body.

Recommended dosage: Up to 250 milligrams twice a day with meals.

Tryptophan. This amino acid encourages the production of serotonin, which has a calming effect on the body. It should be given as a supplement according to body weight. Consult a natural physician to discuss if it is appropriate for your child.

CALMING PRACTICES

Get your child outdoors. Some children are hyperactive due to inactivity. Get your child outside to play. Encourage activities that get the body in motion, such as playing sports and dancing. Limit time in front of the television and on the computer.

Defuse hyperactivity. There are a variety of essential oils with calming effects. Those that are safe for children include lavender, chamomile, cedarwood, and sandalwood, and they all have pleasant-smelling essences. You can use them in a variety of ways.

- Put a few drops into a diffuser or oil ring during study time to help your child focus.
- Mix 30 drops with a cup of distilled water and mist it into the air during times when calm is called for.
- Stir a few drops into your child's bath water at night to help bring on sleep.
- Make or buy a lavender sachet and tuck it into your child's pillow.

WHEN TO CALL THE DOCTOR

If you suspect your child has AD/HD or your school requests that you start your child on Ritalin, see a qualified professional who specializes in behavioral problems in children. Get proactive in your child's care and don't hesitate to ask a lot of questions of both your child's doctor and the school. You should feel comfortable that there is a compelling medical reason for putting your child on psychiatric drugs. Don't give in to pressure.

BACK PAIN

Back pain is the price we pay for our cave-dwelling ancestors' evolutionary rise from four- to two-limb ambulation. We twist, bend, pull, slump, and strain our upright backs in any number of abusive ways, making it the number-one cause of absenteeism on the job.

Most often we bring the problem on ourselves when we don't treat our backs with the respect they deserve. Lack of exercise, poor posture, a bad mattress, or supporting too much weight on the bust or stomach makes our back muscles and ligaments get weak.

Back pain comes in two forms: the acute kind lasts for a few days as a result of stress or strain from overuse. Chronic pain is the persistent and often most painful variety caused by such problems as arthritis, a past injury, a herniated disk, or sciatica.

HOW INJURY HAPPENS

The disks of the spinal cord are fibrous rings surrounding a pulpy core that separate the spine's vertebrae. A disk is herniated when the pulpy material pushes against a root. The most notorious back pain—sciatica, which occurs in the lowest part of the back and causes a pronounced shooting pain down the leg—is a disk pressing the tender sciatic nerve.

Back pain can also signal a problem elsewhere in the body, such as a kidney or bladder problem.

Surgery was once the most popular recommended remedy for chronic back pain, but nowadays even surgeons call for it only as a last-ditch effort. Though there are many

medications to quell the pain and inflammation, there are
natural remedies that can do the same.

RELIEF AT LAST

White willow. Aspirin is one of the most widely used
antidotes for inflammation due to back pain. But you can go
to the direct source of aspirin and sidestep its often harsh
side effects. The active ingredient in aspirin is salicin, which
is found in the bark of the white willow plant. Take it as a
supplement or brew it into a tea.

Recommended dosage: Take one or two capsules a day.

Caution: If you are allergic to aspirin, you probably will
be allergic to white willow as well.

Wintergreen. Oil of wintergreen is a pleasing-smelling
essence that also contains salicin. It is recommended by
aromatherapists as a massage oil to soothe achy backs and
spasms.

Caution: Wintergreen is intended for topical use only, as
ingesting even a small amount is potentially dangerous.

Mint. The mint family contains compounds similar to
menthol and camphor, which are found in over-the-counter
muscle relaxants.

Cayenne. The substance that makes peppers hot is capsaicin, which helps block substance P, the body's main pain
messenger. Look for creams and ointments containing capsaicin and use according to package directions.

Ginger. This strong culinary condiment contains
inflammation-relieving compounds.

Recommended dosage: Two capsules in the form of
dried powder twice a day.

Calcium and magnesium. These two minerals help alleviate muscle spasms. Take it daily in a multivitamin.

Recommended dosage: 250 milligrams of magnesium
and 500 milligrams of calcium a day.

Bromelain. This enzyme, which is a derivative of pineapple, helps ease muscle spasms.

Recommended dosage: 500 milligrams three times a day.

PAY ATTENTION TO PREVENTION

Lose weight. Overweight is a common cause of back pain. Change your diet to natural foods low in calories and fat and you should lose weight gradually.

Practice perfect posture. Stand straight and tall with your weight evenly balanced on both feet. Rotate your shoulders backward as a reminder throughout the day to stand tall.

Sit without slumping. The same rules for standing apply for sitting. During times of pain, you can manage your posture by sitting in a straight chair.

Stay limber. Aerobic and weight-bearing exercise will keep your back strong. Yoga is an excellent exercise to get the back limber and keep it limber.

Lift right. Proper lifting means bending at the knees, not bending over.

WHEN TO CALL THE DOCTOR

If you don't get natural relief for acute pain after several days or relief from chronic pain after two weeks, see your doctor. You should also see your doctor if back pain is accompanied by other symptoms, such as shortness of breath, fever, or pain elsewhere in the body.

BAD BREATH

Bad breath is a lasting impression you don't want to leave. It is generally caused by the buildup of bacteria in the mouth, which can result from poor diet, a long absence between meals, dry mouth, certain medications, and, obviously, a lack of attention to dental hygiene.

Bacteria are also the cause of "morning mouth." During the day, oxygen-rich saliva keeps the mouth acidic, which keeps bacteria at bay. At night, the chemical environment of the mouth turns more alkaline, which attracts bacteria. Get rid of the bacteria and you'll get rid of the bad breath.

If your taste in food leans toward garlic, onions, or other pungent and spicy foods, lingering odor can frequently be part of who you are. These foods contain odor-producing sulfur compounds that permeate not only the mouth, but the bloodstream and lungs as well. It can sometimes take up to 24 hours for the odor to dissipate.

Smoking, alcohol, and coffee can also call unwanted attention to your breath.

It is good hygiene to be mindful of your breath. When a toothbrush or mouthwash are not at hand, there are a number of ways to whisk away unpleasant mouth odor.

HERBAL MOUTH FRESHENERS

Aromatic seeds. Anise, dill, cardamom, and fennel seeds contain compounds that kill bacteria and freshen breath. Pop a few in your mouth and chew.

Clove. Its antibacterial action comes from the substance called eugenol. Clove has a strong taste, so try it one clove at a time.

Parsley. The practice of garnishing a dinner plate with parsley started as a way to provide diners with a natural after-dinner breath cleanser. The cleansing comes from chlorophyll, the pigment that gives parsley its rich green color.

Peppermint. This is the best antidote for bad breath caused by eating garlic, onions, and other pungent spices.

The oils in peppermint travel through your bloodstream, chasing these lingering odors away.

Lemon. Fresh lemon is an antibacterial agent that also helps neutralize acids.

WHEN TO CALL THE DOCTOR

Persistent bad breath is medically called halitosis and can be a sign that something is not right somewhere in the body. Chief among potential problems is periodontitis, a bacteria-causing gum disease that, if not treated, can lead to tooth loss.

If you have bad breath that does not respond to good oral hygiene, you should see your dentist.

BELCHING

A little burp every now and then calls for nothing more than the polite refrain, *excuse me*. But some people are plagued by persistent belching that is more irritating than just a social faux pas.

Belching is the result of built-up air in need of somewhere to go, so it backs up and comes out the mouth. The belly fills up with air because we swallow it, mostly unconsciously as we eat and drink. Swallowing air is all part of the normal digestive process, but sometimes we take in too much air, which causes too much pressure.

We expel gases when we belch, too. Gas is an intestinal by-product of incomplete digestion, which is a common reaction to milk sugar, fat, and fiber in a meal. It can cause discomfort and indigestion.

To squelch excessive belching, try the following.

NATURAL REMEDIES

Ginger. The rhizomes in this herb are good for many kinds of gastrointestinal woes, including belching. Bite into a piece of fresh, peeled gingerroot or take it in capsule form.

Recommended dosage: Take two capsules of powdered ginger before meals.

Seeds. Fennel, anise, and celery seeds are carminative agents, meaning they help expel gas.

Cardamom. Follow meals with a cup of cardamom tea to help aid digestion. Brew one teaspoon of cardamom in a cup of water and steep for ten minutes.

PAY ATTENTION TO PREVENTION

Eat slowly. When you gulp down your food, you swallow excess air.

Go strawless. A straw may seem like the natural solution to airless drinking but it actually causes you to swallow more air. Taking small sips helps, too.

Forego fizzy drinks. Carbonated drinks are full of air bubbles. Same goes for sparkling wine and beer.

Get the air out of your diet. Foods that are aerated, like whipped cream, pancakes, and fluffy eggs are notorious belching agents.

BITES AND STINGS

Life's smallest creatures have a mighty big way of saying hello. They bite or sting and leave a lasting memory of your brief encounter: itching and unsightly welts that will ruin the way you look in a pair of shorts and a tank top.

Mosquitoes, flies, fleas, wasps, and bees are among the most common insects that bite. Fortunately, most insect bites and stings are minor annoyances that go away in a few days. But the itching can feel like torture, and the welts can leave unsightly marks in all the wrong places.

Here's what you can do to get the better of these little buggers without resorting to chemical warfare.

FAST FIRST AID

Soap and water. Certain insects, such as fleas and mosquitoes, can spread disease, so make sure to wash the bite site well with soap and water.

Garlic and onion. These herbs contain enzymes that break down chemical substances that the body releases in response to pain. Make a poultice of pressed fresh garlic and onion skin and apply it to the bite. You can even eat garlic and onion as a means to repel insects.

Essential oils and lemon. Essential oils that help relieve the pain, itching, and swelling of bites and stings include basil, chamomile, bergamot, patchouli, and tea tree. Mix a few drops in a little lemon juice and apply with a cotton ball.

Lavender. Lavender is mild enough to apply full strength. Put a drop or two on a cotton ball and dab it on.

NATURAL REPELLANTS

Citronella. Citronella is commonly sold as an outdoor candle to keep insects away and it is even an ingredient in some commercial repellants. The essential oil itself, however, can be irritating, so you should not apply it to your skin.

Mountain mint. This plant contains pulegone, which acts as a natural insect repellant. (*Pulegium* means flea in Latin.) It can be rubbed directly on the skin.

Anti-insect herbs. Insects just hate the smell of certain herbs. If you like to spend a lot of time in your yard, you can help keep insects away by planting an herb garden containing any of these: lemon thyme, lemon balm, basil, and any member of the mint family.

WHEN TO CALL THE DOCTOR

Not all insect bites are harmless. Ticks are the source of some serious illnesses, such as Lyme disease and Rocky Mountain spotted fever. Also, any harmless bite can turn into an infection. Seek medical help right away if a bite gets hot and painful, if you develop a fever, or if you break out in hives.

Bee stings can be a dangerous allergen to some people. If a bee sting results in wheezing, swelling, tightness in the chest, or any other unusual symptoms, consider it a medical emergency. Any one of these could be a sign of potentially fatal anaphylactic shock.

BRONCHITIS

Cold, flu, or bronchitis—how can you tell? Bronchitis has a calling card: a chest full of mucus that you cough, hack, and bring up in shades of gray or green.

Other symptoms can include fever, chills, tightness in the chest, painful breathing, and shortness of breath.

Bronchitis feels like it's all in your chest but it actually is an inflammation of the bronchial tubes, which connect the trachea, or windpipe, to the lungs.

Attacks of acute bronchitis are common during flu season, when viruses are populating homes, schools, and work places. Most cases, about 90 percent, are viral in origin and will go away on their own in about two weeks.

Chronic bronchitis is more troublesome because it is caused by something in the environment, such as pollution or smoke, that is irritating the airways. It usually develops over time. Smokers, coal miners, and people exposed to dust and dirt are often sufferers of chronic bronchitis. Chronic bronchitis is characterized by persistent coughing and wheezing.

People with chronic bronchitis are at high risk of developing heart disease and more serious lung disease.

Though most cases of bronchitis will clear up on their own, there are natural medicines that will help alleviate the fever, coughing, and general blahs that interfere with life as usual. Here is what you can do to stem the symptoms enough to focus and feel well enough to get through the day.

EASING THE SYMPTOMS

Eucalyptus. To keep mucus flowing, inhale eucalyptus oil, a well-documented natural expectorant. Put a drop or two on a hanky and inhale.

Mullein. Known for its powers to protect the respiratory system, mullein is another natural expectorant that will help loosen phlegm. It will also help ease the muscle spasms that trigger a cough.

Recommended dosage: Take 2 capsules a day or mix 1 teaspoon of dried leaves in a cup of water and steep. Drink 3 times a day.

English plantain. This well-known cough suppressant can be enjoyed as a tea. Mix one teaspoon of the dried herb in a cup of boiling water and steep.

Marshmallow. This herb is a natural demulcent, meaning it helps soothe sore mucous membranes. Drink it in a tea.

Echinacea. This popular choice for respiratory health is believed to help stimulate infection-fighting white blood cells.

Recommended dosage: Take 500 milligrams in capsule form three times a day.

Vitamin C. Studies show that people hospitalized for bronchitis recover faster when they take vitamin C supplements.

Recommended dosage: Take 1,000 milligrams three times a day.

Zinc. Proper immune function and tissue repair depend on adequate levels of zinc in the body. Suck on zinc lozenges according to package directions.

N-acetylcysteine. This amino acid, commonly called NAC, can help thin and loosen mucus.

Recommended dosage: 300 milligrams twice a day.

R-lipoic acid. This nutrient with antibiotic properties is important to the health of the respiratory system.

Recommended dosage: 100 milligrams three times a day at mealtime.

IN THE KITCHEN

Eat hot foods. Put chili, hot salsas—anything with chili pepper—on your menu. It will help break up congestion and thin mucus.

Drink orange juice. Lots of liquids are good for keeping mucus flowing, so fortify yourself with extra vitamin C by drinking orange juice.

Make a pot of chicken soup. It's an old-fashioned remedy with modern scientific validity. Eating a hot bowl of chicken soup helps stimulate mucus flow and ease congestion. Make sure it contains garlic, onion, cayenne pepper, and thyme—all of which help fight respiratory invaders.

Avoid milk products. Milk contains lactalbumin, which stimulates the production of mucus.

WHEN TO CALL THE DOCTOR

Most cases of bronchitis clear up on their own. Sometimes, however, bronchitis can mask or lead to pneumonia. If this is the case, you want to get medical treatment as soon as possible.

Those at risk for pneumonia are the elderly and people who have asthma or any other respiratory illness, heart disease, or a compromised immune system.

Call your doctor if you experience a fever of 103 degrees or higher, extreme lethargy, wheezing, or difficulty breathing. Also, call your doctor if any of the following occur.

- Your cough is so persistent it keeps you up at night and interferes with daytime activities.
- Symptoms last more than a week and mucus becomes darker in color.
- You have difficulty breathing.

BRUISES

Call it a badge of courage, a symbol of honor, or a sign of stupidity. Whatever you call it, it will give you something to talk about for quite a while, because the bigger the bruise, the longer it will take to heal.

A bruise, or black and blue mark, is a sign of trauma to the skin caused by a fall, blow, or collision with a door, piece of furniture, or other hard object. The impact causes capillaries, tiny microscopic blood vessels just beneath the skin, to break, bleed, and clot, causing the skin to turn a dark shade of blue. As the blood starts to reabsorb, the skin will go through a rainbow of colors—purple, brown, and yellow—before it eventually disappears.

Black and blue marks can be very painful, though it may not be as painful to the skin as it is to your ego. The memory of the incident will fade, as surely as the discoloration to your skin.

FIRST-AID ACTION

Cold. Before doing anything, apply a cold compress or ice bag to a bruise to prevent swelling and severe coloration.

Apply at 15-minute intervals for the first several hours, then every hour for the first 24 hours.

Hot and cold. Try heat and cold compresses for the next 24 hours. You also can soothe the bruise with any of the following.

Pineapple. You're more likely to see a boxer walking around with a steak on a black eye than pineapple, but he'd be better off with a pineapple ring. Pineapple contains bromelain, a sulphur-containing enzyme that has been proven effective in speeding the healing of black and blue marks. Bromelain comes in capsules and tablets.

Recommended dosage: 1,200 MCU (milk-clotting units) throughout the day.

Arnica. Also known as mountain daisy, Arnica is a popular homeopathic remedy for bruised skin because it contains pain-relieving and antiseptic qualities. Commercial arnica ointments are sold in health food stores. Look for a product containing 15 percent arnica oil and use it according to package directions.

Comfrey. Its name is so close to comfort, especially for the skin. Comfrey contains a compound called allantoin, which promotes skin repair. Soak a cloth in comfrey tea and apply it to the bruise.

Parsley. This remedy is an old wive's tale with anecdotal validity. Press a bunch of fresh parsley and place it against the bruise. Tie it with a loose bandage to keep it in place.

Vitamin C. This antioxidant vitamin is important to skin health because the body uses it to produce collagen, a protein that helps keep connective tissue and blood vessels strong. Vitamin C has also been shown to help wound healing.

Recommended dosage: Take 500 milligrams three times a day.

Vitamin K. This nutrient is essential for blood to clot. Make sure that your multivitamin contains vitamin K.

Recommended dosage: To help heal a bruise, take 2 milligrams daily.

Green leafy vegetables. Increase your intake of leafy greens during the healing process. They are good sources of vitamins C and K.

Bioflavonoids. Sometimes referred to as vitamin P, bioflavonoids are nutrients found in the pigment of various plants that help reduce tissue damage.

Recommended dosage: 500 milligrams three times a day.

WHEN TO CALL THE DOCTOR

If you find your skin is bruising easily when it never did before without an obvious cause, you should see your doctor. Bruising can be a sign of disease or an imbalance of clotting factors in your blood chemistry.

BURNS

Burns hurt—*a lot.* Even a split-second encounter with the handle of a pot simmering on the stove is a sharp reminder of just how sensitive, and delicate, the skin can be.

Burns can occur in an infinite number of ways: flame, hot coil, steam, hot liquids, electricity, chemicals, and the sun are among them. The severity of a burn depends on the source of the burn, the place and percentage of the body burned, and the depth of the burn.

Burns are classified as first, second, or third degree. First-degree burns are the type usually encountered in the kitchen that cause red and painful skin. Second-degree burns will blister and ooze. Third-degree burns can appear charred or milky white in color. They may not hurt if nerve endings have been destroyed. Third-degree burns are always medical emergencies.

These remedies are intended only for first-degree and certain second-degree burns.

Aloe. This is more than a folk remedy. The gel of the aloe vera plant has been used for centuries to treat burns and other wounds. Aloe vera is a succulent plant that is easy to grow. Many people keep one on the kitchen window so it will be handy in the event of an encounter with a hot pot or oven. When a burn happens, slice a piece of one of the plant's spiky leaves and let the gel ooze over the burned tissue.

Lavender. Aromatherapists argue that lavender essential oil is as effective as aloe in soothing a burn. Keep a vial on your kitchen windowsill next to your aloe vera plant.

Gotu kola. Triterpenic acid is a compound in the gota kola plant that has been found to hasten healing time and prevent scarring in severe burns.

Recommended dosage: 30 to 60 milligrams a day of gotu kola containing triterpenic acid.

Vitamin C. There is evidence that vitamin C, when taken along with gotu kola, can increase its effectiveness.

Vitamin E. When the burn starts to heal, break open a vitamin E capsule and let the gel run over the wound. It not only helps promote faster healing, but it feels good, too.

Zinc. Zinc helps promote wound healing. When recovering from a burn, make sure to eat foods rich in zinc. For insurance, you should also take zinc supplements.

Recommended dosage: 30 milligrams a day.

Propolis. A resin similar to bee pollen, propolis can be found as a spray, salve, or tincture. Use according to package directions.

WHEN TO CALL THE DOCTOR

Consider a burn a medical emergency requiring a trip to the doctor or hospital in the following cases.

- The burn oozes and/or gets worse instead of better.
- The burn occurs on the face, near the eyes, or in the pelvic area.
- The burn is caused by a chemical, electricity, or prolonged contact with a hot surface.

BURSITIS AND TENDINITIS

Skier's knee, runner's ankle, tennis elbow, and housemaid's knee are nicknames for the skin afflictions known as bursitis and tendinitis—names that are strongly suggestive of their root cause: repetitive motion.

Collectively known as repetitive motion syndrome, bursitis and tendinitis are actually two distinct conditions that share similar symptoms and treatments.

Bursitis is an inflammation of the bursae, tiny fluid-filled sacs that provide a cushion between muscle and bone. Tendinitis is inflammation in or around the tendon, the tough cords that attach muscle to bone. Both conditions cause inflammation and swelling that make even the smallest effort to move the affected area hurt like the dickens. A not-so-obvious difference is that bursitis produces a dull pain, while tendinitis produces sharp pain. Bursitis commonly affects the shoulders, elbows, hips, knees, and the joints in the feet and hands. Tendinitis usually affects the shoulder, wrists, heel, and elbow.

Both conditions come in two forms: acute, meaning the discomfort only lasts a few days, and chronic, meaning it comes and goes and is tough to get rid of.

The goal in all cases is to relieve pain and reduce inflammation, and make them go away permanently. Doctors commonly do this with nonsteroidal anti-inflammatory drugs, such as aspirin, or powerful prescription medications called corticosteroids. Instead of going for the heavy-artillery drugs, try these natural solutions.

NATURAL PAIN RELIEF

RICE. Your first line of remedial action should be RICE—rest, ice, compression, and elevation.

White willow. The bark of the white willow plant contains salicylates, a natural precursor of aspirin. Hence its nickname, herbal aspirin. For tender joint pain, herbalists recommend a willow tea. Take two teaspoons of dried herb per cup of water and bring it to a boil. Steep for 20 minutes. Relax, elevate your limb, and sip a cup three times a day.

Arnica. This homeopathic remedy with anti-inflammatory qualities comes in a rub designed to treat bursitislike pain. Look for it in health food stores and follow the packaging directions.

Cassia oil. This essential oil, which is imported from China, contains properties that reduce inflammation and ease sore muscles. A relative of cinnamon (and similar in taste), cassia oil is the active ingredient in Tiger Rub, an emollient available in health food stores.

Boswellia. This extract from the frankincense tree helps reduce the production of pain-producing substances. Start out at the highest dose and gradually reduce it as the pain subsides.

Recommended dosage: 400 milligrams three times a day.

Bromelain. Herbalists recommend bromelain, a natural anti-inflammatory agent found in pineapple, for acute pain.

Recommended dosage: 500 milligrams three times a day without food.

Curcumin. This compound found in turmeric, a popular

hot spice commonly used in Indian dishes, has healing qualities similar to cortisone.

Recommended dosage: 400 to 500 milligrams three times a day.

KITCHEN'S PAIN CHASERS

Eat pineapple. A common folk tale circulating in athletic circles says that eating pineapple before and after a workout helps protect tendons and joints. This most likely stems from the fact that pineapple contains enzymes that break down protein. One such enzyme is bromelain.

Get your vitamin C. Vitamin C assists collagen production, which is essential for the formation of tendon and bursal tissues. Eat plenty of foods containing vitamin C. Also, consider taking 1,000 milligrams of vitamin C a day while you're recovering.

Magnesium. This mineral is important to healthy muscles, bones, and connective tissue.

CANCER

The human body is in a constant state of change. At this very moment, millions of cells in your body are dying and being replaced by new ones. It could be taking place in your muscles, your bones, your pancreas, or possibly all three. This is all part of the normal cycle of life.

The rate at which cells replicate varies from organ to organ and tissue to tissue. For example, the cells that line the small intestine replace themselves every few days. Other cells stick around for a long time. Pancreatic cells replicate about once a year. Cells also have the ability to replicate on short notice as a result of damage or injury.

They'll reproduce fast, then slow down to their natural pace once the healing process is over.

New cells are formed through a process called cell division—a process controlled by the genes.

HOW HEALTHY CELLS BECOME CANCER CELLS

Genes are codes within a cell that tell cells how to behave. Genes dictate coded messages through the many different proteins that form the building blocks of cells. Normal genes automatically know when it is time to start cell division and stop replication. Sometimes, however, a gene gets damaged, or mutated—perhaps as a result of an inherited weakness or an environmental invader. When a cell mutates, it loses its ability to communicate properly, causing it to multiply and divide at an unusually fast rate. Eventually these newly formed cells cluster together, forming a tumor. Doctors also have a special name for mutated cells: oncogenes, or cancer genes.

Some lumps of cells are benign, meaning they are not cancerous and are usually harmless. Others are malignant and continue to grow, robbing healthy cells of nutrients in the process and interfering with the body's normal functions. A tumor that goes undetected will continue to grow and its cells can spread to other parts of the body, where new tumors begin. This process is called metastasis.

Keep in mind that it is not easy for a normal cell to become cancerous. This is because cells also contain genes specifically designed to stop their mutant brethren from sending the message to multiply. These are called tumor suppressor genes.

Mutated cells also have the ability to self-destruct. Or, they may be recognized and killed by an alert immune system. Fortunately, most precancerous cells die before they are able to form a tumor. Only a few actually get away. Also, it can take a long time for mutating cells to grow into a cancerous tumor—this is the reason why the rate of cancer increases with age.

MANY AND DIFFERENT CANCERS

Though all cancer involves the uncontrolled growth of cells, cancer is actually an umbrella term for more than 100 different diseases. There are four main categories of cancer.

- Carcinoma of the skin, mucous membranes, glands, or other organs.
- Leukemia, which attacks the blood.
- Sarcoma of the muscles, connective tissues, or bones.
- Lymphoma, cancer of the lymphatic system.

Areas of the body where malignant tumors most commonly develop are the bone marrow, breasts, colon, liver, lungs, lymphatic system, ovaries, pancreas, prostate gland, skin, stomach, and uterus.

While many cancers can be treated successfully, the sad fact remains that cancer is the second most common cause of death, after heart disease, in the United States.

Despite its prevalence, the exact cause of cancer remains a mystery. While experts believe heredity is a factor, it is not the only one. There is strong evidence that environmental factors—such as exposure to tobacco smoke, radiation, asbestos, toxic wastes, certain lifestyles, and nutritional substances—are to blame, meaning that certain kinds of cancer are largely preventable.

THE ROLE OF NATURAL MEDICINE

It is beyond the scope of this book to offer a thorough investigation of all the possible and potential treatments for cancer, natural or otherwise. Natural medicine's most important voice in cancer, as it is with all disease, is about prevention. But even here the possibilities are vast and could fill an entire book.

The best overall preventive tactic is to live a healthy lifestyle that encompasses a whole-foods diet, regular exercise, clean air, stress control, and a strong support system. There are also specific supplements, foods, and lifestyle practices that may offer added protection as well. These are some of them.

TOPS IN NUTRITION

Phytonutrients. More than a decade ago scientists started to find that plant foods contain naturally occurring nutrients more powerful than vitamins and minerals at protecting health and fighting disease. To date, more than 800 different phytonutrients have been identified and scientists believe that there are thousands yet to be discovered.

A lot of the ongoing research, however, is focused on several different classes of phytonutrients that possess substances with even greater antioxidant powers than found in the essential vitamins A, C, E, and the mineral selenium. This is significant in the fight against cancer because antioxidants are our number-one nutritional defense against mutating precancerous cells. Scientists are also studying other classes of phytonutrients for their ability to rid the body of harmful cancer-causing toxins.

Phytonutrients with antioxidant action include the following.

- Carotene
- Flavonoids
- Lignans
- Lutein
- Lycopene

- Phenols
- Tannins

Phytonutrients that help rid the body of toxins are as follows.

- Ellagic acid
- Glucosinolates
- Indoles
- Lignans
- Isothiocyanates
- Limonoids
- Sulforaphane

Phytonutrients come in supplements, but there are many scientists who believe that the only sure way to get their protective and healing benefits is to get them through food.

Beta-carotene. Also known as provitamin A, beta-carotene is what gives deep green and orange fruits and vegetables their rich color. Numerous population studies show that diets rich in beta-carotene are protective against a variety of cancers. Conversely, low blood levels of beta-carotene have been linked to an increased risk of different types of cancer, especially breast, bladder, colon, and lung cancer.

If you do not get a minimum of five servings a day of carotene-rich fruits and vegetables, you should consider a supplement.

Recommended dosage: 25,000 I.U. a day.

Vitamin C. This important antioxidant has been shown to protect against cancer on many levels. It helps prevent genes from forming mutating cells, bolsters the immune system, and is a powerful detoxifier.

Recommended dosage: 500 to 1,000 milligrams a day.

Vitamin D. A 15-nation study has concluded that the incidence of colon and breast cancers would go down if people would get adequate vitamin D, both from the sun and through diet. Research indicates that people who reside north of the equator do not get adequate vitamin D, especially during the winter months.

Recommended dosage: 2,000 I.U. plus 10 to 15 minutes in the sun a day.

Vitamin E. Evidence suggests that vitamin E is the hardest worker when it comes to fighting the oxidative wear and tear that leaves the body vulnerable to carcinogens. Studies have found low levels of vitamin E linked to breast cancer. Vitamin E may also help prevent stomach cancer and other cancers of the gastrointestinal tract by inhibiting the conversion of nitrates in foods to nitrosamines, which are potential carcinogens.

Recommended dosage: 400 I.U. daily.

Selenium. This trace mineral works synergistically with vitamin E to help prevent free-radical damage. Broad-based population studies show that selenium is protective against cancers of the breast, colon, and lung.

Recommended dosage: 200 micrograms a day.

Fish oil. Omega-3 fatty acids found in fatty fish help strengthen the immune system and have been shown to be protective against certain types of cancer. If you do not eat fatty fish at least three times a week, consider taking a fish oil supplement.

Recommended dosage: 500 to 1,000 milligrams a day.

D-glucarate. This phytonutrient is proving to be a powerful detoxifying agent. Preliminary studies in animals show that it helps prevent certain kinds of cancer.

Recommended dosage: 400 milligrams in capsule form a day.

THE CANCER-FIGHTER'S CUPBOARD

Green tea. Evidence of the health and healing potential of green tea continues to mount. At the top of the list is its ability to fight cancer. It has been linked to protection against bladder, breast, colon, liver, lung, prostate, and throat cancers. Studies show that populations that drink green tea on a daily basis have an overall lower incidence of cancer.

Green tea contains several compounds of polyphenols not found in other edible plant substances. For every cup of green tea you drink you will be getting about 100 important polyphenols. If you are not a steady tea drinker, consider taking supplements.

Recommended dosage: 500 milligrams of green tea extract containing at least 80 percent polyphenols a day.

Garlic and onions. This pungent duo, both members of the allicin family, contain a variety of cancer-protecting agents including flavonoids, phenolic acid, antioxidants, and sulphur. Onions are also a unique and rich source of quercitin, a flavonoid that early studies show may help suppress the formation of cancerous tumors. If you shun onions, consider taking quercitin supplements.

Recommended dosage: 500 milligrams three times a day.

Seaweed. It's no coincidence that Japan, the nation that boasts the highest longevity rate in the world, also eats an abundance of seaweed (among other healthful eating practices). Seaweed is one of the most nutritionally dense foods on earth. It is a powerful detoxifier and inhibits the formation of cancerous tumors. New studies show it is protective against certain forms of cancer, including breast and cervical cancer.

Ginseng. Ginsenoside, a compound found in ginseng, is a phytonutrient with steroidlike compounds that has been found to be protective against cancer. In one study, those who took ginsenoside in the form of Panax ginseng had half the risk of cancer than those who did not take the supplement. Panax is Chinese ginseng and has different properties than American ginseng.

Soy. The soybean is a bounty of special cancer-protecting phytonutrients, including isoflavones, phenolic acids, phytosterols, and saponins. Population studies show that people who eat a diet rich in soy have the lowest cancer mortality rates. For example, Chinese women, who eat soy as a staple in the diet, have one-fifth the rate of breast cancer as American women, who eat very little soy. Asian consumption of soy products is 200 percent higher than American consumption.

Turmeric. This popular Indian spice contains curcumin, a potent antioxidant that has been shown to suppress cancer-causing mutagens. Studies show it may have special protective effects against nicotine. Keep a jar in your kitchen cupboard. If you are a smoker or exposed to secondhand smoke, consider taking a curcumin supplement.

Recommended dosage: 500 milligrams of curcumin daily.

CANKER SORES

Whoever coined the medical term *aphthous stomatitis*—fire sore—must have been speaking from experience, because the pinhead-size mouth ulcer delivers crater-size pain.

It's a medical mystery as to what causes mouth ulcers to pop up on the tongue or inside the cheeks and lips or why some people are plagued with them and others aren't. The best guess to date is heredity.

Canker sores are harmless but can last up to a week or more if left to heal on their own—a long time considering every bite and every sip can deliver a searing pain. Remedial action can help clear them up in a day or two.

SORE SOOTHERS

Salt and water. Mix half a teaspoon of salt with half a cup of warm water and swish around the sore for as long as you can take it. Repeat as needed.

Teabag. Apply a slightly warm, wet teabag directly on the sore for several minutes throughout the day as needed. Tea contains tannin, which is a mild astringent.

Cankerroot. American Indians used this herb to heal mouth sores, hence the name. If you can find it, brew it into a tea.

Licorice. This herb contains glycyrrhetinic acid, which scientifically has been found to speed the healing of canker sores. Licorice also contains tannins. Look for lozenges containing deglycyrrhizinated licorice, commonly called DGL.

Recommended dosage: Chew 1 or 2 tablets a day.

Aloe juice. Put on a cotton tip and apply.

Zinc. This mineral promotes wound healing.

Recommended dosage: Take a 30-milligram lozenge a day.

PAY ATTENTION TO PREVENTION

Acidophilus. The live culture in yogurt is a friendly bacterium that will help balance the acidic environment in the mouth. Eat a few tablespoons a day.

Steer clear of certain foods. Eating too many foods high in acid, such as tomatoes, strawberries, and citrus, can bring on an outbreak in some people.

B vitamins and iron. Several studies show a correlation

between canker sores and low stores of iron and vitamin B, especially folate.

WHEN TO CALL THE DOCTOR

If a canker sore or cluster of sores linger for more than a week, contact your doctor or dentist. You may need an antibiotic or a doctor may need to cauterize the sore. In addition, the sharp end of a tooth or another dental problem could aggravate a canker sore and prevent it from healing.

CARPAL TUNNEL SYNDROME

Repeating the same task over and over and over can be dull and boring. It can also be dull and painful.

Carpal tunnel syndrome, also known as repetitive stress injury, came into the common medical lexicon when the word processor, then computer, became the tool of choice in the workplace. It develops over time as a result of repeated stressful movement of the hands and wrist.

Carpal tunnel is a cumulative trauma disorder caused by compression of the medial nerve, which runs from the forearm to the fingertips and lies between the ligaments and bones of the wrist. The medial nerve controls the movements of the fingers and thumbs.

Carpal tunnel is characterized by pain, weakness, numbness, tingling, and burning in the wrist and fingers that often radiate to the forearm and shoulder. It appears in people who use their hands a lot, such as typists, assembly-line workers, keyboard operators, cashiers, knitters, and carpenters. It can also follow a more serious injury to the wrist, or other condition that causes swelling of the tissues in the wrist, such as arthritis.

HELPING THE HAND

Vitamin B6. Therapeutic doses of vitamin B6 are probably the most well-known pain-relief remedy but are also the most controversial. B6 is important for maintaining healthy nerves, but excessive amounts also can cause nerve damage. B6 helps relieve pain associated with carpal tunnel syndrome in some—but not all—patients. Generally, vitamin B6 helps some patients, especially when it is combined with supplements of vitamin B2 and other B vitamins. Doses in the range of 500 to 150 milligrams a day are considered within the safe range. However, you should err on the side of caution and take B6 only with the consent and under the supervision of medical practitioner. Better yet, boost your intake of B6 foods.

Magnesium. This trace mineral is important to healthy nerves. It also helps muscles relax. Eat more magnesium-rich foods and consider a supplement.

Recommended dosage: 300 milligrams twice a day.

Bromelain. This is a protein-dissolving enzyme produced by the pineapple plant that helps relieve pain and inflammation.

Recommended dosage: 250 to 750 milligrams twice daily between meals.

Curcumin. This potent anti-inflammatory, derived from turmeric, is considered a natural alternative to cortisone.

Recommended dosage: 250–500 milligrams a day.

Cayenne. Red pepper contains capsaicin, which is found in commercial pain-relieving ointments. Add a tablespoon of cayenne to a quarter cup of unscented lotion and rub it on your wrists.

PAY ATTENTION TO PREVENTION

Carpal tunnel can be very painful, so the best approach is to prevent it. Here's what you can do.

- Adjust your chair and keyboard so that your arms are bent at a 90-degree angle and your wrists are parallel to the ground when you type.
- Use a contoured or split keyboard designed for your hands to rest in a natural position while you type.
- Take frequent breaks when doing repetitive tasks.
- Do exercises that stretch the arms, wrists, and hands.

WHEN TO CALL THE DOCTOR

Consult your doctor if you continue to experience pain after one month of self-treatment. In some cases, surgery is required to ease the pain.

CATARACTS

Imagine what it's like wearing sunglasses on a cloudy day. That's kind of what the world looks like when you have cataracts.

Cataracts are cloudy spots that film over the normally translucent lens of the eye, causing impaired vision. They can even lead to blindness. Your risk of developing cataracts increases with age but they are not inevitable. Cloudiness of the lens is caused by oxidation, a biochemical process in which free radicals attack and damage the protein structure of the lens. Oxidation is a part of normal everyday living—which is why risk rises with age—but there are lifestyle and environmental factors that can speed it up. Leading factors include excessive and cumulative sun exposure, pollution, smoking, and a diet chronically low in protective antioxidant nutrients. People with diabetes have an increased risk of cataracts. Heredity can also increase risk.

UNPREDICTABLE GROWTH

Cataracts don't always behave in a predictable manner. They can develop quickly or slowly, they can affect one eye or both, and they can progress at different rates from one eye to the other.

Cataracts aren't obvious to the naked eye until advanced stages. But an ophthalmologist can detect early onset using special instruments, which is why routine eye exams are essential.

An estimated 4 million Americans have sight-impairing cataracts, and they are one of the leading causes of blindness in the aged. Medical treatment is surgery. Preventive measures are a much easier route. You can both prevent and help slow the progression of cataracts with antioxidants.

EYE FOOD

The antioxidant formula. Research shows that people with high levels of antioxidants in their blood have a lower risk of developing cataracts. This means eating a diet rich in dark green leafy vegetables and fruits, among other foods. (For a complete list of foods high in these nutrients, see page 90). You can also fortify yourself with the following.

- 500 milligrams of vitamin C
- 400 I.U. of vitamin E
- 15 milligrams of beta-carotene
- 80 milligrams of zinc

Hues of red and blue. Anthocyanins are a pigment that gives the skins of red and blue fruit their distinctive hues. They belong to a class of antioxidant-rich phytonutrients called bioflavonoids. Research shows that the largest concentration of these important antioxidants is found in the skin. This is significant because anthocyanins aim much of their antioxidant action toward the eye. Fruits containing these compounds include blackberries, bilberries, blueberries, cranberries, raspberries, grapes, plums, and wild cherries.

Carrots. Bugs Bunny knows what he is talking about: Carrots are good for the eyes. Carrots are rich in carotenoids, the compounds that give carrots their full-bodied color. More than two dozen studies have shown that a diet rich in carotenoids helps reduce the risk of getting cataracts. Eat plenty of carrots and other carotenoid-rich plant foods, or take a supplement.

Recommended dosage: Take 25,000 I.U. of mixed carotenoid complex twice a day.

Brazil nuts. Studies have found a correlation between low levels of selenium and cataracts. A small handful of Brazil nuts contains more than the Daily Value for the trace mineral selenium. Selenium also helps boost the action of vitamin E, also abundant in Brazil nuts.

Bilberry extract. During the war, British pilots snacked on bilberries before flying night missions to sharpen their night vision. In one study, bilberry extract plus vitamin E stopped progression of cataract formation in 48 out of 50 patients with age-related cataracts.

Recommended dosage: Take 100 to 150 milligrams of bilberry extract three times a day.

WHEN TO CALL THE DOCTOR

Cataracts tend to impair vision gradually, making it difficult to notice slight changes in vision. Regular eye exams are necessary to catch the disease in its early stages, so get an eye examination annually.

Symptoms of more advanced cataracts include dull, fuzzy vision, glare in bright light, double vision, and changes in color vision.

CHAPPED LIPS

Lips are a flaw in an otherwise flawless facial design.

Lips feel and look different than other facial skin because they are thinner and contain more nerve endings, which make them sensitive to touch; they have no melanin, which visually exposes blood vessels and gives them their distinct red color. They also lack protective hair, sweat glands, and body oils, which makes them kissably soft.

And herein lies the flaw. Sweat glands and their naturally occurring oil also regulate temperature, keep skin soft, and help guard against germs. Because they lack sweat glands, lips are vulnerable to parching, peeling, and cracking.

Lips need constant attention and routine protection in order to keep them looking and feeling luscious. Here's what to do.

DAILY LIP SERVICE

Jasmine absolute. The oil from the jasmine flower conditions the lips at the deepest level and feeds emerging cells with its vitamin-rich oil. The oil is so powerful that it has the ability to feed skin robbed of its sweating mechanism. Jasmine contains only infinitesimal amounts of volatile oil, so it is very expensive. Look for lotions containing jasmine absolute, such as Clark's Botanicals Ultra Rich Lip Balm, available online and through select department stores.

Vitamin E. For really sore lips, open a vitamin E capsule and apply as needed.

Lanolin. This inexpensive lubricant helps put moisture back into sore, chapped lips. Look for over-the-counter balms and creams that list lanolin as a key ingredient.

Petroleum jelly. This thick gel is not the best tasting but it is inexpensive and effective.

Combination creams. Bag Balm contains lanolin and petrolatum; Burt's Beeswax Lip Balm also contains coconut oil, almond oil, vitamin E, and comfrey.

PAY ATTENTION TO PREVENTION

Lipstick. Lipstick is moisturizer for the lips. It also protects the lips from the sun.

Sunscreen. The sun will fry your lips, so protect them with a lipstick with a built-in sunscreen. Men should look for clear balms containing sunscreen.

Water. Dry lips can be a sign that you are not drinking enough water. Make sure to get 8 eight-ounce glasses a day.

CHOLESTEROL

Like most things in life, cholesterol isn't all bad. High cholesterol, however, is a different matter. You have to take it seriously because it is a major health threat; it also puts you at risk for heart attack, stroke, and other life-threatening diseases.

Cholesterol isn't all bad because the body requires it for certain basic functions. For example, it forms a protective sheath around nerve fibers and helps manufacture certain hormones. The body, however, doesn't depend on food for cholesterol like it depends on food for vitamins and minerals. The body has the ability to produce all the cholesterol it needs on its own. This is why we can end up in cholesterol trouble.

All cholesterol activity takes place in the liver, where it is processed into fatty acids. Substances called low-density lipoproteins (LDL) pick up the fatty acids and send them into the bloodstream for deposit in needed cells. If too much cholesterol goes out, other substances called high-density lipoproteins (HDL) pick up the excess and take it back to the liver where it is broken down and excreted from the body.

Normally, LDL and HDL do a pretty good job of balancing cholesterol, but when the bloodstream is flowing with more cholesterol than HDL can handle, the excess needs a place to go—and it usually goes into the artery walls where it oxidizes and hardens. As cholesterol deposits build up, arteries get narrower and narrower—the perfect setup for a heart attack or stroke.

BALANCING THE HIGH AND LOW

As scientists accumulate more data on cholesterol, the more conservative they get as to what is considered a healthy level. The current recommendation is to get your LDL cholesterol as low and it can go and keep your HDL high. Women should shoot for an HDL of 50 and higher and men 45 and higher; the higher the better. LDL should be lower than 100. Doctors consider a high LDL level a risk even if HDL is high. Total cholesterol isn't considered as important, although the rule of thumb is to keep levels below 200.

Some people struggle with high cholesterol no matter what they eat because their bodies manufacture too much. This tendency is often inherited. There is also an indication that eating dietary cholesterol stokes the body's natural cholesterol-manufacturing process.

Long ago the strategy to lower cholesterol was to banish or severely limit your intake of cholesterol-containing foods. (Cholesterol is only found in animal foods.) But researchers have discovered there are a lot of dietary ways to manipulate HDL, LDL, and total cholesterol. There are foods that can help reduce total cholesterol, but there are also foods that have the special ability to boost protective HDL and lower artery-clogging LDL.

CHOLESTEROL CUTTERS

Olive oil. Fat takes the rap as the cholesterol king and for good reason. But not all fat is bad. The fat that contributes to cholesterol buildup is saturated fat, the kind concentrated in butter, meat, and other animal-based products. Monounsaturated fat, however, is a different story. Studies show that monos have the ability to reduce LDL and raise HDL. Olive oil is almost 100 percent monounsaturated fat.

Recommended dosage: 1 to 3 tablespoons a day.

Other oils. Other mono oils to include in your diet are avocado oil, almond oil, and canola oil.

Almonds and walnuts. One study found that adding three ounces of nuts per day to an otherwise low-fat diet brought down total and LDL cholesterol

Recommended dosage: A handful of almonds and/or walnuts a day.

Garlic. Studies show that eating garlic on a regular basis can lower total and LDL cholesterol without affecting HDL. It can also help break up substances that form clots. Eating a clove or more a day has been shown to reduce total cholesterol 10 to 25 percent. Garlic tablets can also have the same effect.

Recommended dosage: Eat a minimum of a clove of garlic a day or take up to 500 milligrams as a supplement a day.

Soluble fiber. Soluble fiber plays a unique role in your cholesterol count. The digestive process is dependent on cholesterol because the liver uses it to make bile acids. When soluble fiber comes in contact with bile acids it absorbs them and takes them along for the ride outside of the body. As a result, the liver must gather more cholesterol to make more bile acids. Studies show this has a significant effect on reducing total cholesterol.

Soluble fiber is found in oats, beans, barley, fruit, and flaxseed.

Recommended dosage: 10 to 25 grams of soluble fiber a day.

Pectin. This is a soluble fiber found in fruit, most notably apples and pears.

Soy. An analysis of 38 studies found that people who ate soy foods as a protein substitute for meat had overall lower cholesterol and triglyceride levels than meat eaters. Researchers chalk up soy's special cholesterol-lowering ability to its rich isoflavone content.

Policosanol. Studies show that policosanol, a fatty acid supplement, can produce results similar to cholesterol-lowering drugs.

Recommended dosage: 10 to 20 milligrams a day.

ANTIOXIDANT ACTION

Fruits and vegetables. Fruits and vegetables with deep hues of green, blue, orange, and red are a sign that they are loaded with antioxidants. Antioxidants with special cholesterol-reducing attributes are beta-carotene, vitamin C, vitamin E, and selenium. Eat five to nine servings a day plus an antioxidant supplement.

Recommended dosage: Take a high-potency antioxidant formula as directed.

Blueberries. The blues are a powerhouse of pterostilbene, a compound that has the ability to activate the cellular structure that helps lower cholesterol. Studies show that blueberries can be as effective as certain drugs at lowering cholesterol.

Onions. Onions contain three unique compounds that are proven cholesterol busters: Flavonol, hydroxybenzoic acid, and quercitin.

Fish oil. Studies have found that fish oil supplements help reduce both cholesterol and triglyceride levels.

Recommended dosage: Fish oil containing up to 450 milligrams of EPA and 350 milligrams of DHA a day.

COLDS AND FLU

Dare to find someone who can say they've never had a cold or the flu. It just isn't going to happen. In fact, you can consider yourself lucky to get through a year without catching one or the other.

Colds and flu bugs are hard to duck because there are more than 200 different viruses that cause them and new ones are sprouting all the time. Building an immune defense to each and every one is darn near impossible because the immune system tends to suppress one virus at a time. (This is why children are more susceptible to sickness than adults.)

The common cold and typical flu are a lot alike because they share similar symptoms. With the flu, though, you'll also experience fever, more pronounced aches and pains, and more fatigue. But either one is going to make you feel lousy.

Since a cure for the common cold and flu still evades modern science, the best you can do is try to suppress the symptoms. Here are some natural remedies that don't have the side effects of over-the-counter drugs.

NATURAL COLD REMEDIES

Zinc. At the first sign of a cold or flu, pop a zinc lozenge into your mouth and suck on it. Studies have found zinc lozenges can curtail a cold by three or four days.

Recommended dosage: Take according to package directions.

Vitamin C. Since 1970, more than 20 studies have found

that vitamin C helps decrease the duration and severity of cold and flu symptoms.

Recommended dosage: 1,000 milligrams three or four times daily, as tolerated.

Astragalus. Studies have found this traditional Chinese herb effective at reducing the duration and severity of cold and flu symptoms. Astragalus works by stimulating virus-destroying white blood cells and enhancing the production of interferon, a natural compound that fights viruses.

Recommended dosage: Take 250 to 500 milligrams of dried root capsules two to three times daily with food.

Echinacea. More than 350 studies have examined the immune-enhancing properties of echinacea. While not all of the studies have had positive results, the majority suggest that echinacea helps reduce the duration and severity of symptoms.

Recommended dosage: 500 milligrams three times a day.

Goldenseal. If you have a lot of mucus, take goldenseal in combination with echinacea. This herb contains alkaloids that dry up mucus flow.

Recommended dosage: Take 500 milligrams along with echinacea three times a day.

Ginger. For chills and a sore throat, drink up to four cups of ginger tea a day. Ginger can also help stop a cough.

Slippery elm. Brew a tea made with this herb to suppress a cough and soothe a sore throat. Or look for a cough drop containing slippery elm.

Chicken soup. It's an old-wives tale no longer. Studies show that a hot bowl of chicken soup can help break up congestion and diminish other symptoms of cold and flu. Make sure the soup contains potent amounts of viral-fighting garlic and onions.

PAY ATTENTION TO PREVENTION

Cold and flu viruses can spread like wildfire, so the best way to avoid catching what's going around is to take measures to bolster your immune system and keep your distance from those already infected with a virus. To this end, you should do the following.

- Eat a healthy diet containing vitamin C-rich foods.
- Take immune-enhancing herbs and supplements, especially vitamin C.
- Wash your hands frequently.

WHEN TO CALL THE DOCTOR

Most colds and flu don't require a doctor's care, but sometimes these illnesses can lead to something more serious, like pneumonia. If you develop a fever of 103, or your symptoms don't abate or get worse after 10 days or so, you should call your primary-care physician.

COLD SORES

What do nearly 90 percent of Americans have in common? Cold sores—or at least the virus that causes them.

A cold sore, also known as a fever blister, is caused by the highly contagious herpes simplex virus that lies dormant in a nerve until some outside force—such as cold, the sun, or stress—triggers it and it shows up as a sore, fluid-filled large blister somewhere on the face, usually the lip. The virus is so common that most people who have it were exposed before the age of five. Only about a third of those who have the virus never experience an outbreak.

Most people are forewarned of a pending attack by a

tingling and burning sensation about three days before an outbreak. By this time, it is too late to avoid it, but there are things you can do to ease the soreness and speed healing.

L-lysine. This amino acid has been found to both speed healing and suppress outbreaks.

Recommended dosage: 2,000 to 3,000 milligrams to speed healing and 500 to 1,000 milligrams for prevention.

Lemon balm tea. Herbalists credit lemon balm, also known as Melissa, with having special anti-herpes properties. Take 4 teaspoons of the dried herb and brew it in a cup of hot water. Apply the tea directly to the sore using a cotton ball.

Tea tree. Mix equal parts of tea tree essential oil and olive oil and dab on the blister several times a day.

Echinacea. Studies show echinacea has ample antiviral action to fight an attack.

Recommended dosage: 300 milligrams four times a day.

PAY ATTENTION TO PREVENTION

Acidophilus. The active culture found in yogurt has been found effective at suppressing the virus. Eat several tablespoons a day.

Zinc. This trace mineral helps strengthen the mouth tissue, making it harder for a blister to take hold.

Avoid arginine. The herpes simplex virus is partial to the amino acid arginine, which is found in foods such as beer, cola, chocolate, and nuts.

CONSTIPATION

It could be caused by something you ate—or something you didn't eat. It could be a side effect of a new medication, or your body's rebellion to stress or travel. Whatever the cause, constipation will make you feel decidedly irregular.

Constipation is not defined by how frequently you move your bowels. In fact, there is no definition of "normal." But it is not normal to get bloated, pass gas, and strain unsuccessfully as a result of stools too dry to pass.

Everyone gets constipated every now and then, but chronic constipation can lead to digestive and intestinal woes. It can also cause hemorrhoids and varicose veins.

The most common cause of constipation is insufficient intake of fiber and fluids. Iron tablets, antidepressants, and some painkillers can also cause constipation. Constipation is also common during pregnancy.

A MOVEABLE FEAST

The last thing you want to do to relieve constipation is take a chemical-based laxative. They not only treat you unkindly but you can grow dependent on them. Rather, reach for a natural laxative that will bring relief in a more natural way.

Psyllium. This is Mother Nature's most effective laxative because it contains a bulk-forming fiber called mucilage. Psyllium is the active ingredient in over-the-counter laxative formulas. You can find them in pleasant-tasting flavors. Take as directed daily to both relieve and prevent constipation.

Aloe vera. This herb contains anthraquione, a powerful compound that behaves like a laxative. It is most effective taken as a juice.

Recommended dosage: One-half cup aloe vera juice in the morning and evening.

Fenugreek. Like psyllium, this herb contains mucilage. Swallow several fenugreek seeds with a large glass of water twice a day.

Flaxseed. If you don't like the taste of fenugreek, try flaxseed. Make sure to drink it with plenty of water.

Prunes. Prunes are high in fiber and contain a compound that makes them the most stool-stimulating fiber food. Eat the fruit or drink a glass of prune juice.

PAY ATTENTION TO PREVENTION

A few healthy dietary changes can make chronic constipation a thing of the past.

- Eat at least five servings of high-fiber foods every day, particularly wheat bran.
- Drink plenty of fluids—at least 8 glasses a day.
- Get regular exercise, which helps stimulate the bowels.

DANDRUFF

We're willing to put up with a lot of life's little annoyances, but dandruff is not one of them.

People hate dandruff; some even consider it a social stigma. Which is probably why the shampoo industry is spending millions of research dollars seeking a dandruff shampoo that really works.

There is nothing unclean about dandruff. It's just residue from the skin's natural process of shedding old skin to make room for new. Usually the scalp sheds skin invisibly. The shedding and flaking that characterize dandruff is a sign that the scalp is replenishing cells a lot faster than normal. Why this happens is unclear, but people with a naturally oily scalp are more prone to dandruff. The problem is remarkably common: as many as one out of five people has dandruff.

HOW TO SCALE BACK

Biotin. Biotin is a B vitamin important to healthy hair and nails. Dry, flaky skin is a major sign of a biotin deficiency. Foods containing biotin include soybeans, barley, oats, and avocado. If these foods are not part of your diet, consider a biotin supplement.

Recommended dosage: 6 milligrams of biotin a day.

Tea tree. The oil from this plant contains terpenes, an antisepticlike substance that can penetrate the top layers of the scalp.

Recommended dosage: Add 10 drops of tea tree oil to a 10-ounce bottle of regular shampoo.

Comfrey. Allantoin, the healing chemical in this herb, has anti-dandruff properties. Look for shampoos containing comfrey or add a few drops of the essential oil to your shampoo and conditioner.

DEPRESSION

I'm so depressed. How often have you heard or even said this sad refrain? Probably quite a bit. That's because it is an expression that covers a spectrum of negative emotions, from having a blue Monday, to a sense of dread, to profound sorrow.

True depression, however, is more than feeling down this week and back in the game the next. It is a lack of interest in life and the inability to deal with normal everyday living. It involves feelings of worthlessness, pessimism, sadness, loneliness, and disinterest in anything or anyone. It can trigger exaggerated negative reactions totally out of proportion to the cause. With clinical depression, these feelings linger for weeks or months and ultimately become incapacitating.

AN EXPLAINABLE CAUSE

Some people inherit a tendency toward depression or an imbalance in brain chemistry that leads to depression. It can result from dealing with a chronic problem or illness—your own or someone else's—such as stroke, chronic fatigue, cancer, thyroid disease, alcoholism, or drug abuse. Some drugs can cause depression, too.

Whatever the cause, most experts now recognize depression as an organic illness that has both physical and psychological triggers. Most people cannot just "snap out of it," no matter how hard they try, meaning professional counseling is crucial to recovery. But there are things you can do on your own to cure the occasional blue mood.

GOOD MOOD MAKERS

St. John's Wort. Modern scientific studies now validate this old folk remedy for depression. St. John's wort contains the chemical hypericin, which has been shown to be even more powerful than some antidepressant drugs—and without side effects. While many people have reported positive effects within the first two weeks, it can take three to four weeks until you notice a significant change.

Recommended dosage: 250 to 300 milligrams of standardized form 0.3% hypericin two to three times a day.

SAMe. S-adenosyl-L-methionine is a substance found in every single cell. It involves some 40 biological processes, including the brain chemicals responsible for elevating mood. Like St. John's wort, SAMe is also has been clinically proven to be as effective as prescription antidepressants. SAMe works best in the presence of B vitamins, so take it along with a B complex vitamin.

Recommended dosage: Up to 1,600 milligrams a day.

B Vitamins. The B's, particularly vitamins B6, B12, and

folic acid, promote a healthy central nervous system. Eat plenty of B-rich foods in addition to taking a B-complex supplement.

Recommended dosage: 50 milligrams of B complex once or twice a day.

5-HTP. 5-hydroxytryptophan is an amino acid involved in the production of the brain chemical serotonin. Low levels of serotonin have been linked to depression. This, too, should be taken with a B-complex vitamin.

Recommended dosage: 100 milligrams three times a day.

WHEN TO CALL THE DOCTOR

It can be difficult to tell the difference between sadness and clinical depression. If you have any of these symptoms, discuss them with your doctor.

- Changes in sleep (either insomnia or sleepiness)
- Changes in weight and eating habits (either weight gain or weight loss)
- Loss of sexual desire
- Chronic fatigue or tiredness
- Low self-esteem or self-worth
- Loss of productivity at work, home, or school
- Inability to concentrate or think clearly
- Withdrawal or isolation
- Loss of interest in activities that were once enjoyable
- Frequent weeping or sobbing
- Thoughts of suicide or death

DIABETES

Diabetes is the fastest growing health problem in America—so much so that doctors have coined terms for its warning signs. One is called "pre-diabetes," a sign that blood sugar levels are at the near-danger level. The other is "diabesity," suggestive of the root cause for the alarming climb in the incidence of this disease.

Obesity and diabetes go hand in hand. And they are both serious business.

A BALANCING ACT

Diabetes is a life-altering diagnosis. It is forced entry into a life that revolves around insulin and blood sugar control.

The disease is characterized by elevated blood sugar levels, and high blood sugar puts pressure on and can damage the pancreas, nerves, and blood vessels. Over a period of time, this can lead to a number of other health problems, including blindness, infections, kidney problems, stroke, and heart disease. Low blood sugar can cause fatigue, lack of concentration, and confusion. If blood levels drop too low—even for a few minutes—it can cause unconsciousness, coma, and even death.

Type II diabetes most frequently is caused by poor dietary choices that cause surges in insulin, the hormone that regulates blood sugar. This taxes the pancreas, where insulin is produced. Over time, the stress damages the pancreas to the point that it can no longer produce and regulate insulin properly.

Type I diabetes used to be known as juvenile diabetes, because it is most frequently diagnosed at a very early age. People with type I produce no insulin and are dependent on daily injections of synthetic hormone. There is an inherited tendency to both type I and type II diabetes.

The good thing about type II diabetes is that it is not only controllable, it is preventable. There is also convincing evidence that it can be reversed.

SUGAR SOLUTIONS

Chromium. This mineral improves glucose tolerance. Chromium makes insulin about ten times more efficient at processing sugar, so less insulin is needed to do the job. Unfortunately, chromium levels tend to decrease with age. Nearly twenty controlled studies have demonstrated a positive effect for chromium in the treatment of diabetes. Most of the studies were performed in patients with type II, or non-insulin-dependent diabetes. In addition to eating foods high in chromium, you should take a daily supplement.

Recommended dosage: 600–1,000 micrograms of chromium daily.

Fenugreek. Fifty percent of fenugreek seed is composed of a soluble fiber called mucilage, which helps control blood sugar. Researchers have been successful using 15 to 100 grams of fenugreek powder daily to treat people with non-insulin-dependent diabetes. Fenugreek should only be taken with the guidance of a medical professional.

Recommended dosage: Up to 1,000 micrograms a day.

Biotin. This B vitamin helps enhance insulin sensitivity and regulate blood sugar. In one study, 8 milligrams of biotin twice daily resulted in significant reduction in fasting blood sugar levels and improved blood glucose control in type I diabetics. In a study of type II diabetics, similar effects were noted with 9 milligrams of biotin daily.

Recommended dosage: 9 to 16 milligrams a day, under a doctor's supervision.

Magnesium. Many people with diabetes have low levels of magnesium, a mineral that is important to insulin production.

Recommended dosage: 300 to 400 milligrams a day.

Manganese. This is another mineral that tends to be low in people with diabetes.

Recommended dosage: 30 milligrams a day.

Vitamin C. This antioxidant will help guard you against complications from diabetes.

Recommended dosage: 1,000 to 3,000 milligrams throughout the day.

Garlic. Garlic helps stabilize blood sugar and is a potent protector against heart disease, a major threat to people with diabetes. Make garlic part of your daily diet or take supplements.

Recommended dosage: 400 milligrams as a supplement daily.

PAY ATTENTION TO PREVENTION

The following lifestyle practices will help keep diabetes at bay.

- Lose weight if you are 20 or more pounds overweight.
- Follow a diet low in saturated fat and refined sugar.
- Eat complex carbohydrates, the kind found in whole grains, beans, and vegetables.
- Limit your intake of fruit to only a few pieces a day.
- Get in the habit of regular exercise, meaning no less than three times a week. Studies show that vigorous exercise can lower the risk of developing type II diabetes by one-third. In fact, many experts consider exercise the most effective way to prevent non-insulin-dependent diabetes.

WHEN TO CALL THE DOCTOR

A fasting blood glucose test should be part of your annual physical. The symptoms of diabetes are not always noticeable in the early stages. The signs of type II diabetes—thirst, drowsiness, obesity, fatigue, tingling or numbness in the feet, blurred vision, and itching—often go unrecognized for years before being properly diagnosed. The symptoms of type I diabetes—excessive thirst, frequent urination, dry mouth, blurred vision, and frequent infections—often develop rapidly. If you experience any of the warning signs, contact your doctor immediately.

DIARRHEA

Diarrhea is good. It's a sign that your body's defense mechanism is working its best to get rid of the nasty something that has invaded your digestive system.

The thought that diarrhea is good for you may not sound very comforting to you right now, but it's the reason doctors usually recommend toughing it out instead of trying to make it stop.

Keep in mind that diarrhea is not a disease; rather it is a symptom of something your body doesn't like—be it a virus, bacteria, protozoa, or spoiled food—or something it can't tolerate, such as lactose, too much fiber, too much sugar, or just too much partying. Diarrhea can also be the unfortunate reminder that you aren't being thoughtful enough about what you're eating and drinking when you are on vacation in a foreign land.

Sometimes diarrhea can be a side effect to a drug or a part of living life with a chronic health problem, such as Crohn's disease or ulcerative colitis.

Even though you should let nature take its course, there is action you can take to make the going less tough.

STEMMING THE FLOW

Lots of liquids. Diarrhea causes the body to lose a great deal of water and essential nutrients, so keep yourself hydrated by drinking plenty of liquids, including water, vegetable juice, and broth. Drinking milk or soft drinks is not a good idea.

Tea. The tannin in plain black tea will help soothe intestinal tissue. Green tea is just as good. Drink up to five cups a day while diarrhea is active.

Carrot. Strained carrots is a well-known home remedy for diarrhea in babies, but it works just as well for adults. Carrots contain pectin, a soluble fiber that adds bulk to stools. It also helps soothe the digestive system. Eat half a cup every hour until symptoms ease.

Apple. Apple is another rich source of pectin. This is why applesauce is such a good home remedy.

Bilberry. Dried bilberry contains both pectin and tannins.

Recommended dosage: 160 milligrams twice a day.

Probiotics. Diarrhea takes the good bacteria out of your system as well as the bad. You can replace the bacterial balance in your system by eating yogurt containing live cultures of acidophilus. Eat yogurt or take acidophilus as a supplement.

Recommended dosage: 1 teaspoon acidophilus powder in 8 ounces of distilled water twice daily.

PAY ATTENTION TO PREVENTION

Wash and wash. The substances that cause us to eat something we shouldn't aren't visible to the naked eye so diarrhea isn't totally avoidable. However, you can help reduce the risk by being vigilant about washing your hands before, during, and after contact with food. Also, wash fruits and vegetables before cooking or eating them raw.

Garlic. Before traveling to a foreign country, fortify your digestive system by taking garlic supplements four to six weeks prior to the trip. Garlic is a strong antibacterial and antiviral agent. Take it while you are traveling as well.

WHEN TO CALL THE DOCTOR

A serious consequence of diarrhea is dehydration, especially in a child. If you see any of these signs, contact the doctor right away.

- Infrequent urination
- Dark or concentrated urine
- Loss of skin elasticity
- Lethargy

DIVERTICULAR DISEASE

No one ever heard of diverticulitis 100 years ago. Sure, people ate the meat of cows, pigs, and wild animals. But they also ate plenty of foods of the earth—vegetables, fruits, and whole grains. Then in the name of progress, some forward-thinking industrialist comes up with an invention that split the fiber in grains and sugar and made them white.

People indulged in these refined foods heartily, even though it sometimes resulted in constipation and other bathroom complaints. What they didn't realize was what the lack of fiber was doing to their colons.

INSIDE THE COLON

As you age and the decades pass, a low-fiber diet causes the taut and smooth colon to weaken and form tiny pockets and bulges. When this happens, you have diverticular disease: you just don't know it because it isn't causing you any trouble—yet. Sometimes, though, the tiny pockets can get lodged with food particles, causing the colon to become inflamed and infected. This you will notice: pain, nausea, diarrhea, and constipation are signs of diverticulitis.

Diverticulitis is serious because it can lead to potentially life-threatening peritonitis if it is not medically treated right away with antibiotics.

Diverticular disease, however, doesn't have to get this far. You may not be able to make the tiny pockets disappear but you can help the colon work the way it is supposed to by adding more fiber to your diet.

HIGH FIBER ACTS

Flax. Flax is a fiber so good for the colon that doctors in Germany use flaxseed as a treatment for diverticulitis. Take flax daily, according to directions.

Psyllium. This fiber is the active ingredient in most natural laxative supplements. It will help keep stools soft and help prevent particulates from wedging in the diverticula.

Recommended dosage: Take daily as directed on package directions.

Wheat. Forego white bread and grains for whole-wheat varieties.

Slippery elm. Its fibrous bark powder is used by herbalists to treat diverticulitis. Eat it regularly mixed with water like you would oatmeal.

Water. Fiber depends on plenty of water for bulk to pass smooth, easy stools. Make sure you drink plenty of water every day.

PAY ATTENTION TO PREVENTION

Eating a diet high in fiber and getting regular exercise will promote good bowel habits and minimize your risk of developing diverticulitis.

WHEN TO CALL THE DOCTOR

If you have persistent and severe pain in the lower abdomen and develop a fever, contact your doctor immediately.

You may have an infection within the digestive tract that could require prompt medical attention.

EARACHE

The ear canal is to the body what a border is to a country: a no-trespass zone for unwanted aliens. And like any country, your success at defending your ear canal from foreign invaders depends on your body's defense system.

Children are most vulnerable to earaches and ear infections because their ear canals are so small and their tiny bodies are still building an immune defense. But adults can get ear pain, too.

When something like water, smoke, or another allergen invades the ear canal, the middle ear starts secreting mucus, which can block the Eustachian tubes that lead to the throat. This is why you instinctively will open your mouth in all kinds of contorted ways to try to make your ears "pop."

In fact, many ear problems begin in the Eustachian tube. The Eustachian tube is the passageway for the bacteria that causes the common childhood middle ear infection known as *otitis media*. People with shorter Eustachian tubes are more vulnerable to ear infections—which is why children will "outgrow" their tendency toward ear infections.

Swimmer's ear, or *otitis externa*, is an infection of the outer ear. It is characterized by itching or tingling outside the ear, sometimes with a yellowish discharge. If your ear hurts when you gently pull it and wiggle it, chances are good you have an outer-ear infection.

FIRST AID FOR THE EARS

Kali Mur. Homeopathic physicians use this form of sea salt to treat fluid in the ear. Look for Kali Mur 6X and take according to package directions.

Ferrum phosphoricum. This is a form of iron that homeopathic physicians use to treat ear infections in children. Take according to package directions.

Echinacea. This herb is noted for its antibacterial action and ability to boost the immune system.

Recommended dosage: 1 dose three times a day for 3 days, followed by 1 dose once a day for 4 more days.

Ephedra. This herb is the natural equivalent of the over-the-counter decongestant Sudafed. Action comes from ephedrine and pseudoephedrine that can help drain fluid from the middle ear. Ephedra should not be given to children and should be taken by adults with caution.

Recommended dosage: 1 teaspoon a day brewed as a tea.

Garlic. Herbalists recommend garlic for ear infections because of its antifungal and antibacterial powers. It is most effective as an eardrop.

Recommended dosage: 1 or 2 drops of garlic oil in the ear once or twice a day.

WHEN TO CALL THE DOCTOR

If your or your child's ear problem does not respond to natural remedies and symptoms get worse, call your doctor. Antibiotic treatment may be required. An untreated ear infection can lead to hearing loss.

If you experience ear pain and a yellowish or bloody discharge from the ear, call your physician. Your eardrum may have ruptured. The eardrum will heal (in fact, the rupture is part of the body's healing process), but your doctor may need to prescribe antibiotics to speed the healing and prevent additional infection.

ECZEMA

Eczema is dry skin gone to extremes. It shows itself as scaly, red patches on the skin, usually on the elbows, knees, and hands.

It is also *very* itchy, and the more you scratch the worse it gets. It can even ooze and become crusty.

Why some people are plagued with eczema is a question not even a dermatologist can answer for certain. But doctors do know that people with eczema have supersensitive skin that acts in very unpredictable ways.

In some people, eczema is an allergic response to anything from food, wool, and perfume to pollen, metal, and chemicals in detergents and soap. Doctors call this atopic, or contact, dermatitis. Other people seem to get an outbreak for no reason at all. Eczema also tends to run in families. Babies sometimes show eczemalike rashes, but they usually go away as they grow. True eczema can come and go for a lifetime.

The most common trait shared among people with eczema is very dry skin. They also tend to have thicker than normal skin with a limited capacity to hold water. This may be due to the fact that people with eczema seem to have trouble processing certain fatty acids. Natural therapy is aimed at restoring a nutritional balance.

HELP FOR SENSITIVE SKIN

Evening primrose oil. Physicians in Great Britain and Germany use evening primrose oil to treat eczema. It contains a highly useable form of gammalinolenic acid, or GLA, an amino acid that tends to be low in people with eczema. It can be applied to sore skin or taken as a capsule.

Recommended dosage: Two 500-milligram capsules three times daily.

Omega-3. The omega-3 essential fatty acid found in fish oil and flaxseed is involved in suppressing chemical reactions that release histamines in response to allergens.

Recommended dosage: 1.8 milligrams of fish oil or 2 tablespoons of flaxseed oil a day.

Vitamin E. This oily antioxidant promotes skin healing and prevents oxidation of essential fatty acids.

Recommended dosage: 400 I.U. a day.

Zinc. This mineral is important to healthy skin. Some people with eczema have low levels of zinc in the blood. Have a blood test to find out if you are low in zinc, as excess zinc can cause a copper deficiency.

Recommended dosage: 30 milligrams twice a day.

Calendula. The essential oil soothes and helps heal inflamed skin. Apply directly to the skin and rub in.

Oatmeal. A relaxing way to soothe sore, itchy skin is to take an oatmeal bath. Look for colloidal oatmeal for a bath and follow the directions.

PAY ATTENTION TO PREVENTION

If you have sensitive skin, you need to avoid everything that irritates the skin or causes allergic reactions. Some suggestions.

- Wear cotton instead of wool, silk, or synthetics.
- Avoid long showers and baths, which will dry out your skin.
- Moisturize after a shower while the skin is still moist.
- Wear rubber gloves when handing solvents or cleaning supplies.
- If you swim in a chlorinated pool, rinse thoroughly to remove all traces of chemicals.

EMPHYSEMA

Emphysema is a disease that gives true meaning to the expression, *you leave me breathless*. Why? Because it is a debilitating lung disease of slow suffocation.

Emphysema is the aggressive assault of white blood cells on alveoli, the tiny air sacs in the lungs. Damaged alveoli lose their ability to send life-giving oxygen into the bloodstream and carbon dioxide out of it. As a result, the lungs function poorly, making breathing difficult. As the disease progresses, it literally leaves you gasping for air. In advanced stages, a person may be required to depend on an oxygen tube to breathe. It causes such weakness that even walking across the room becomes impossible.

The sad thing about emphysema is that it is almost totally preventable. Smoking is the cause of 99 percent of emphysema cases, according to statistics. Long-term exposure to harmful air particles and chemical vapors cause the other cases.

Emphysema starts as chronic bronchitis. The combination of emphysema and chronic bronchitis is known as chronic obstructive pulmonary disease.

Emphysema is irreversible and doctors find it difficult to manage. Treatment is aimed at thinning mucus or clearing it from the lungs. There are some natural remedies that can help this process.

MAKING ROOM FOR OXYGEN

N-acetylcysteine. NAC is a derivative of the amino acid cysteine. It has several functions, including as a mucolytic, meaning it has the ability to thin and move mucus out of the lungs.

Recommended dosage: 200 milligrams three times a day.

Mullein. This herb also acts as a mucolytic. Brew 1 teaspoon of dried crushed mullein leaves in a cup of hot water and steep. Drink as a tea two or three times a day.

Vitamin C. This antioxidant is famous for its ability to defend the respiratory system.

Recommended dosage: 500 milligrams twice a day.

Cayenne. The capsaicin in red pepper is an expectorant that also helps protect the lungs at the cellular level. Put several drops in a glass of water and drink it.

Eucalyptus. When inhaled, eucalyptus stimulates airflow.

Green tea. This mighty antioxidant contains theophylline, a compound that can help move mucus up from deep within the lungs. Drink several cups a day.

PROTECT THE LUNGS

Breathing and exerting yourself becomes a real challenge when you have emphysema. These practices will help you breathe easier.

Avoid cold air. It can make the airways spasm.

Exercise moderately. It helps strengthen breathing muscles.

Breathe like a baby. Belly breathing, or diaphragmmatic breathing, is the most efficient way to get oxygen.

Drink plenty of fluids. It helps thin mucus.

Avoid air pollution. If this means moving out of a congested city, do so.

Avoid smoke and smokers. This should go without saying.

PAY ATTENTION TO PREVENTION

Smoking is an addiction that is difficult to break. Sometimes, though, the right incentive comes along that makes quitting stick. Try this one: Every time you get the urge to smoke hold your breath for 30 seconds. This is what every breath can feel like when you have emphysema.

If you don't smoke, you have a 99 percent chance that you'll never get emphysema.

ENDOMETRIOSIS

It is not out of the ordinary for a woman to experience some discomfort during the first few days of her menstrual cycle. Aching, cramping, bloating, and even a bad mood are all part of life for many women during the reproductive years. But a normal menstrual cycle does not wreak havoc and disrupt everyday living month after month. If this is the case with you, you've got to think: *Could it be endometriosis?*

Endometriosis is a condition in which tissue closely resembling the lining of the uterus (the endometrium) grows outside the uterus, invading the abdominal cavity and affecting, and sometimes even attaching to, other organs. Telltale symptoms of endometriosis include increasingly painful periods, tenderness and swelling in the lower abdomen that can start weeks before menstruation, pain in the groin and lower back, pain during urination and bowel movements, and sudden, piercing pain during sex. In some cases endometriosis can cause infertility.

OUT-OF-CONTROL TISSUE

During a normal menstrual cycle, shed tissue flows through the cervix, into the vagina, and out of the body. During the menstrual cycle, it is normal for small amounts of endometrial tissue to push through the fallopian tubes and into the abdomen. This doesn't cause a problem because the immune system zaps it. Or, at least, that is what is supposed to happen. For women with endometriosis, the immune system isn't effective and tissue proliferates and thickens in response to the female hormone estrogen just as it does inside the uterus. It is estimated that between 2 and 5 percent of women between the ages of 25 and 40 end up with endometriosis.

Women with endometriosis tend to have lower levels of natural killer cells and high levels of estrogen. The root cause of endometriosis is a medical mystery, but many theories abound. There is evidence linking it to estrogenlike environmental pollutants that weaken and compromise the immune system. These pollutants include pesticides, herbicides, hormones injected into cattle raised for butchering, home cleaning supplies, and plastics.

There is also evidence of a heredity link. The risk of developing endometriosis is above average for women who have a mother and/or a sister with the condition. There is also a belief that the risk goes up the longer a women puts off motherhood.

Endometriosis is hard to manage and can result in surgical removal of the uterus. There are, however, natural steps you can take to both reduce the symptoms and the odds of getting the disease.

THE DIET CONNECTION

Organics. Eat fruits and vegetables that are free of herbicides and insecticides. Avoid red meat, but if you can't, eat only meat products that are certified to be organic.

Soy. Soybeans contain genistein and diadzein, two estrogenlike plant compounds that prevent the body from absorbing harmful forms of estrogen circulating in the bloodstream.

Indoles. This phytochemical helps the detoxification of estrogen from the liver. Indoles are found in fruits and vegetables such as apples, broccoli, Brussels sprouts, and cauliflower. Or take a supplement.

Recommended dosage: 300 milligrams of indole-3 carbinol a day.

Fiber. Foods high in fiber, most notably whole grains, beans, and vegetables, help balance the bacterial environment involved in the metabolism of estrogen.

Flaxseed. Lignans, which are abundant in flaxseed, are substances that have been found to help control growth of endometrial tissue. Or take flaxseed oil.

Recommended dosage: 1 to 2 tablespoons of flaxseed oil a day.

GETTING HERBAL

Raspberry. Herbalists recommended red raspberry tea to help uterine inflammation and pain. Drink up to three cups a day.

Chasteberry. Also known as vitex, this herb helps balance estrogen levels. You should not take chasteberry if you are on birth control pills.

Recommended dosage: 160 milligrams of 0.6 percent aucubin standardized extract a day.

Dandelion root. This herb helps improve liver detoxification.

Recommended dosage: 300 milligrams a day.

TAKE YOUR VITAMINS

B complex. B vitamins play an important role in estrogen metabolism.

Recommended dosage: 50 milligrams twice a day.

Vitamin C. This is the workhorse of the immune system. Take as much as your body will tolerate.

Vitamin E. This antioxidant helps fight inflammation and controls estrogen metabolism.

Recommended dosage: 400 I.U. twice a day.

Iron. The heavy menstrual cycles that are part and parcel of endometriosis could be depleting your iron stores. Talk to your doctor about getting a blood test to check your iron levels. As insurance, make sure to eat plenty of iron-rich foods. However, do not take iron supplements without knowing for sure that they are necessary.

Multivitamin. Look for a high-potency multivitamin formula designed for women.

PAY ATTENTION TO PREVENTION

In addition to eating as described above, you should take measures to avoid environmental pollutants to the extent that it is possible. One measure that is easy to take is to read labels carefully on detergents and cleaning supplies that you use in your household.

You should also get muscle-building exercise. Research shows that a higher muscle-to-body-fat ratio helps reduce blood levels of estrogen. One study found that women who exercise regularly have a reduced risk of developing endometriosis.

Some doctors also suggest avoiding tampons in order to keep menstrual flow free and unobstructed. It's been suggested that tampon use can increase the risk of getting endometriosis.

WHEN TO CALL THE DOCTOR

Though the degree of pain characteristic of endometriosis varies from woman to woman, it generally causes enough pain and pressure to signal that something is not as nature intended. Don't delay seeing your doctor. The sooner you get the condition diagnosed, the better your chances of keeping it in check and avoiding complications that could lead to surgery.

ERECTILE DYSFUNCTION

The night to remember turned into one that you'd rather forget. Only you can't. You know it happens to *every* man sooner or later, but it is different when it happens to *you*.

The occasional inability to perform in the bedroom is a normal and inevitable part of the aging process. As a man ages, the speed of sexual response slows and the intensity of orgasm declines. This is due to a drop in testosterone levels, and a decrease in blood circulating to the penis.

For some men, though, lack of an erection is more than an occasional problem. When a man cannot get or keep an erection, the problem is called impotence, or erectile dysfunction (ED).

To achieve an erection, there must be cooperation among blood vessels, nerves, and tissues. Interference can be caused by both mental and physical factors. Common physical causes include lack of adequate circulation due to artery disease, diabetes, drug abuse, alcoholism, and diseases that affect the nervous system. Common psychological causes include depression, anxiety, stress, and boredom. Certain medications, including tranquilizers, diuretics, antidepressants, and blood pressure drugs can also cause ED.

The first thing to do when you experience erectile dysfunction is to see your doctor to rule out any serious medical condition. After that, there are several herbs and supplements that can help give your arousal a boost.

LOVE POTIONS

Ginkgo. This well-known mental booster can improve the memory in more than your brain.

Recommended dosage: Take 60 to 240 milligrams a day.

Ginseng. This herb is revered in China for its ability to improve sexual function in men. Make sure to get the Asian variety, called panax ginseng.

Recommended dosage: Take 100 milligrams twice a day.

Zinc. This mineral is important to male sexual function because it is essential to the synthesis of the male hormone testosterone. Zinc supplements can cause a copper deficiency, so you'll need to take a copper supplement, too.

Recommended dosage: Take 30 milligrams twice daily and 3 milligrams of copper.

DHEA. Studies show that some men troubled with potency problems have low levels of dehydroepiandrosterone. DHEA levels decrease with age. Get your DHEA level checked before taking a supplement.

Recommended dosage: 25 to 50 milligrams a day.

Ashwaganda. This is the Ayurvedic solution to male potency problems.

Recommended dosage: Take 1,000 milligrams three times a day.

Oatstraw. This South African herb is associated with potency.

Recommended dosage: Take 300 milligrams three times a day.

Vitamin A. This vitamin is essential to the production of sex hormones. Take a high-potency multivitamin–mineral supplement containing vitamin A.

PAY ATTENTION TO PREVENTION

Being in good physical condition can improve potency as well as overall health. Eat a well-balanced diet, and get regular exercise. Avoid alcohol, which can cause temporary impotence.

When making love, take your time, relax, and enjoy some foreplay. Have intercourse more often, since testosterone levels remain higher in men who have sex more frequently.

WHEN TO CALL THE DOCTOR

Impotence shows up at the least convenient times—and with no warning or invitation. A single episode should not be cause for alarm, but a pattern of difficulty maintaining an erection merits a discussion with a medical professional to rule out physical problems.

If natural remedies don't help and your doctor can't find a physical basis for the problem, contact a psychologist or mental health professional. Statistics indicate that therapy can help in four out of five cases of psychologically based impotence.

FATIGUE

Keeping pace in a fast-paced world can be, well, fatiguing. And we all seem to be caught up in it. Fatigue is the nation's No. 1 health complaint.

Doctors used to have a pat answer for it: get plenty of rest, eat a well-balanced diet, and get plenty of exercise. Now they might add, *get rid of the stress.*

Chronic tiredness is a common consequence of living a double life (parent and professional), being the caretaker of both the young and the old, overpromising your valuable time to others, or, so to speak, habitually burning the candle at both ends.

Relentless fatigue can also have an underlying organic cause. Fatigue can be a sign of undiagnosed anemia, diabetes, heart disease, depression, sleep apnea, or any number of conditions. It can be the side effect of a drug, restless sleep, family problems, or tension on the job.

Fatigue can even be a disease in and of itself.

WHEN IT'S CHRONIC

In 1988, the Centers for Disease Control established criteria for a syndrome of symptoms that literally were dragging thousands of people to the doctor. They named it chronic fatigue syndrome (CFS). It's also been called yuppie flu.

If you have CFS, you feel more than just utterly tired. CFS is also characterized by low-grade fever, swollen lymph nodes, muscle weakness, headache, muscle and joint pain, sore throat, depression, and loss of concentration.

The cause of chronic fatigue syndrome is uncertain and diagnosis can be difficult, since the symptoms are similar to other conditions, such as fibromyalgia.

A chief suspect, however, is the Epstein-Barr virus (EBV), which is a member of a larger group of herpes viruses. EBV is suspect because, like other viruses in the herpes group, it remains dormant until it is activated by a weakened immune system. There are many ways the immune system can become impaired: stress, poor diet, insufficient sleep, vitamin deficiency, smoking, alcohol or drug use—things that make you fatigued.

Whatever the cause, fatigue doesn't have to be a life sentence. There are certain supplements that can give your energy level and your immune system a real lift.

MOST HELPFUL SUPPLEMENTS

Magnesium. A deficiency in magnesium can mimic the symptoms of CFS, and many people with CFS are low in magnesium. Magnesium deficiency is common among women and the elderly. Studies of people with chronic fatigue have shown that magnesium supplementation significantly improves energy levels, emotional states and pain.

Recommended dosage: Take 250 milligrams as magnesium citrate or aspirate three times daily.

Ginseng. Both Asian and Siberian ginseng are considered a tonic for chronic tiredness. Ginseng also been clinically proven to strengthen the immune system. Steep one teaspoon of dried herb in a cup of boiling water and drink as a tea. Or take a supplement.

Recommended dosage: 100 to 200 milligrams of dried powdered extract a day.

DHEA. Dehydroepiandrosterone is an important human hormone that declines with age. DHEA is important to energy production and stress reduction, among other things. Low DHEA levels have been associated with the development of age-related diseases. DHEA should only be taken if your doctor has tested you and determined that your levels are low.

Recommended dosage: 5 to 25 milligrams a day.

CoQ10. Coenzyme Q10 is an essential component of the mitochondria, the energy-producing unit of the human cell. CoQ10 levels also decline with age. A blood test will determine if levels are low.

Recommended dosage: 100 milligrams twice a day.

Tyrosine. This amino acid, which is involved in nearly all cell structures, helps stimulate energy-producing neurotransmitters.

Recommended dosage: Take 50 milligrams per pound of body weight twice a day.

Wheatgrass. Advocates of juicing recommend wheatgrass juice as a cure for fatigue.

Eucalyptus. Aromatherapists recommend eucalyptus

essential oil for a quick hit of energy. Just put a drop on a tissue and breathe it in deeply.

LIFESTYLE FACTORS

Exercise. They say it takes money to make money. Well, the same can be said for exercise. You'll have more physical energy if you get out and exercise three to five times a week. Try brisk walking every day at lunch.

Cut the fat. Too much fat in the diet will make you sluggish.

Sleep well. It's hard to feel energetic when you don't get enough sleep. If you have a hard time sleeping, check out the remedies for insomnia on page 165.

WHEN TO CALL THE DOCTOR

Fatigue is a symptom, not a disease. If you are feeling habitually tired for no explainable reason, you should see your doctor.

FIBROCYSTIC BREAST DISEASE

Lumpy breasts are normal. About half of all women have them—clusters of lumps or bumps in one or both breasts that feel like a bunch of small grapes just under the skin.

Lumpy breasts, in fact, wouldn't be a problem at all if they weren't so painful to so many women, especially around the time of menstruation. Doctors call this condition fibrocystic breast disease (FBD), an umbrella term describing any benign (noncancerous) condition that affects the breast.

Lumpy breasts are caused by the enlargement of glandular tissue. Why this happens isn't clear but it is related to fluctuations of the hormones estrogen and progesterone during the menstrual cycle.

The lumps, or cysts, move freely in the breast, are either firm or soft, and may change in size. Pain results as the cysts fill with fluid and the tissue around them becomes thick, placing pressure on the surrounding area. This fluid is normally reabsorbed by the breast tissue, but as a woman ages the ability of the lymph system to absorb the fluid decreases, and cysts remain.

Fibrocystic breast disease is often a complaint associated with premenstrual syndrome (PMS). If you have symptoms of PMS as well as fibrocystic breasts, the treatment options for PMS on page 200 may be more helpful. If fibrocystic breast disease is your primary complaint, try these options.

LUMPS WITHOUT PAIN

Cut the stimulants. The pain associated with FBD is compounded by methylxanthine, the stimulant found in coffee, tea, cola, chocolate, and medications that contain caffeine. Studies show that when women cut caffeine-containing food and drink from their diets, the pain abates or goes away.

Evening primrose oil. Doctors in the United Kingdom prescribe this essential fatty acid as a treatment for the pain and discomfort of FBD.

Recommended dosage: Take 2 capsules three times daily.

Vitamin E. Several studies have found that vitamin E oil also reduces symptoms.

Recommended dosage: Take 800 I.U. daily.

Acidophilus. The culture found in yogurt promotes the excretion of excess estrogen.

Recommended dosage: Take 1 tablespoon liquid extract or 2 tablespoons powder in cool liquid once a day.

Chasteberry. This herb has a natural hormone-balancing effect on the body.

Recommended dosage: Take 40 drops liquid extract or one capsule daily in the morning.

WHEN TO CALL THE DOCTOR

Anytime you find a lump or change in breast tissue, call your doctor right away. Do not try to diagnose fibrocystic breast disease. Do not delay.

FIBROMYALGIA

Mystery pain.

It's about as good an explanation that you're going to get for this condition—actually a constellation of symptoms—coined from the Greek *fibro*, meaning muscle, and *myalgia*, meaning pain.

It's a diagnosis given when virtually everything else has been ruled out. Scientists have yet to figure out what causes fibromyalgia but they do know that the pain is very real—some 6 million Americans are afflicted with what is described as an "energy-depleting, painful-all-over feeling." For many people, the pain is debilitating.

Though no cause has been found, most doctors agree that there is something not right in the body that prevents the mitochondria, the energy center of the human cell, from producing enough energy to fuel the muscles. The result is muscle pain, usually in the upper part of the body, and overwhelming fatigue that can cascade into any number of other symptoms, such as insomnia, headaches, and even depression. In fact, it is akin to chronic fatigue syndrome, which also has doctors baffled.

A BODY OUT OF BALANCE

Theories suggest that the root cause of fibromyalgia is an imbalance somewhere in the body. For example, people with fibromyalgia generally have low levels of serotonin, the hormone known as a pain messenger. A deficiency of magnesium, which can cause achy joints, has also been linked to the condition. There is also a belief that people with fibromyalgia have high levels of toxins in the blood.

The search for a cure has been as elusive as the search for a cause but many people have found relief from these natural remedies.

SUPPRESSING THE PAIN

5-HTP. Hydroxytryptophan is an amino acid involved in the production of serotonin.

Recommended dosage: Take 50 to 100 milligrams three times a day.

Magnesium. One study found that people taking daily magnesium supplements experienced significant improvement in the amount and the severity of muscle pain.

Recommended dosage: Take 150 to 250 milligrams three times daily.

Black cohosh. This herb has anti-inflammatory qualities and also helps relax muscles. Its hormone-balancing effect may be particularly helpful to women.

Recommended dosage: 80 milligrams a day.

Cayenne. Capsaicin, the active ingredient that puts the fire in cayenne pepper, is well known for its ability to help relieve muscular pain when used topically.

Recommended dosage: Look for a lotion containing 0.025 to 0.075 percent capsaicin and use as directed.

SAMe. S-adenosyl-L-methionine is a naturally occurring substance in cells that decreases with age. It is involved in several crucial chemical reactions in the body. At least four clinical studies have found that SAMe produces excellent results in reducing both the number of pain-producing trigger points and helps improve overall mood.

Recommended dosage: Take up to two 500-milligram capsules daily.

Multiple vitamin. Make sure you're getting all the proper nutrients in your diet by taking a high-potency multivitamin.

Detox. You can help cleanse the body of toxins with a three-day fast in which you take nothing except water and unsweetened fruit juices. This is advised only for people who are otherwise healthy and should be done with the guidance of a natural physician or nutritionist with expertise in detoxification programs.

Milk thistle. This herb supports detoxification. Look for the herb with 80 to 85 percent silymarin extract.

Recommended dosage: Take 250 milligrams three times a day.

WHEN TO SEE THE DOCTOR

A physician should check out any unexplainable chronic pain.

The pain known as fibromyalgia is generally found in several of 18 specific body parts, such as the base of the skull and neck, shoulders, back, and inside the elbows and knees. Doctors call them tender points and they are usually felt on both sides of the body.

Fibromyalgia can be a difficult diagnosis because all other diseases have to be ruled out first.

If you experience chronic fatigue and pain, consult your doctor and schedule a complete physical.

FLATULENCE

Passing gas is normal but that doesn't make it acceptable. Like certain other bodily functions, rules of etiquette apply.

The average person passes gas from 10 to 20 times a day with only a rare embarrassing moment. For others, though, flatulence gives new meaning to the term "cramping your social style."

EMISSIONS CONTROL

Gas forms when undigested starches pass from the small intestine and get trapped in the large intestine and bowel, where resident bacteria ferment them. When excess gas builds up, the bowel has to let it go, and it aims for the closest exit way.

These starches, of course, are carbohydrates and the most notorious among them is beans. Black beans, soybeans, limas, and other legumes are high in two specific carbohydrates, raffinose and stachyose, which the body cannot digest. Some people have digestive tracts that can't tolerate lactose, an enzyme found in milk. Artificial sweeteners, fatty foods, deep fried foods, spicy foods, and fermented foods, such as sauerkraut, can also create intestinal chaos. It also is not unusual to experience excess gas when switching to a healthy eating style, because it means you're eating more complex carbohydrates. Combining spicy or acidic foods with dairy products or sugary foods also can cause flatulence.

GAS GUZZLERS

Activated charcoal. This is the best-known, old-fashioned remedy for gas. It is available in most drugstores. Take it according to package directions.

Fennel seeds. Fennel is a carminative, meaning it contains compounds that break up gas-forming action in your bowel. Chew on a few fennel seeds whenever you feel gassy. Or chew on some seeds after a heavy meal to help prevent gas.

Caraway. If you don't like the licorice taste of fennel, try caraway seeds. It has the same effect. Another carminative is cloves.

Peppermint. All members of the mint family have carminative action but peppermint has been used to relieve gas for centuries. Chew on some leaves or drink it in a tea.

Probiotics. Eat a cup of yogurt containing active acidophilus cultures. Probiotics work by normalizing the good and bad bacteria in your body.

Papaya. This tropical fruit contains a substance called papain that helps aid the digestion process. Eat some fresh fruit, drink a glass of papaya juice, or take enzyme tablets.

Recommended dosage: Take 1 to 2 enzyme tablets when needed.

PAY ATTENTION TO PREVENTION

You can control excess gas to a great degree by paying attention to what you eat and how you eat. Be mindful of these tips.

- Chew food thoroughly. It helps digestion and also cuts down on the amount of air you swallow.
- Soak beans in water overnight, then replenish with fresh water before cooking. This helps get rid of some of the gas-producing enzymes in beans.
- Cut down on sugar and fatty foods.
- Avoid foods and drinks containing the artificial sweeteners sorbitol, xylitol, and mannitol.
- If you're switching to a healthy diet high in complex carbohydrates, do so gradually.

GALLSTONES

Gallstones are unpredictable. These rock-hard structures can be smaller than a pea or larger than an egg. They can sit quietly and not cause any trouble or they can block the bile duct and become inflamed, resulting in severe pain in the upper right abdomen. The pain is often accompanied by fever, nausea, and vomiting.

Gallbladder disease is serious business. Untreated, gallbladder inflammation (also called *cholecystitis*) can be life threatening. If a gallstone blocks the bile duct, bile can back up in the system, causing the skin and whites of the eyes to turn yellow with jaundice and the urine to turn dark brown.

These complications arise from problems with the concentration of bile, the yellowish substance the body uses to digest fat. The liver produces bile (which consists of cholesterol, bile salts, and lecithin, among other substances), and any surplus is stored in the gallbladder, a small organ nestled under the liver. If the bile in the gallbladder becomes too concentrated, the cholesterol can crystallize, forming gallstones.

While 80 percent of all gallstones are composed primarily of cholesterol, they can also be formed of pure bile or mixtures of bile, cholesterol, and calcium.

WHO'S AT RISK

Women tend to develop gallbladder disease more often than men; as many as one out of four women over age 55 has gallstones. Extra pounds put you at extra risk of developing gallstones; people more than 20 percent overweight double their risk of developing gallbladder disease.

Other risk factors include a high-fat and high-sugar diet, rapid weight loss, lack of exercise, diabetes, hypertension, and estrogen replacement therapy (the estrogen increases the cholesterol levels in the bile).

Chronic gallbladder disease sometimes necessitates the surgical removal of the gallbladder (a procedure known as a cholecystectomy), but many people can control the disease by making dietary changes and using nutritional supplements.

WHAT GALLSTONES?

If you've had a gallbladder attack you can help prevent it from happening again with any of these supplements that help increase bile flow and dissolve gallstones.

Milk Thistle. Contains the active ingredient silymarin.

Recommended dosage: Take 600 milligrams (standardized to 70 to 80 percent silymarin content) a day.

Dandelion. Well known as "liver tonic."

Recommended dosage: Take 500 milligrams three times a day with meals.

Curcumin. This is the active ingredient in the herb turmeric, which gives curries their distinctive flavor. Eat healthy doses of this herb in curry dishes or take an herbal supplement.

Recommended dosage: Take a capsule containing 150 milligrams of curcumin three times a day with meals.

Peppermint. Herbalists have been using members of the mint family to treat gallstones for centuries.

Recommended dosage: Take 1 to 2 capsules containing 0.2 milliliters of peppermint volatile oil three times daily between meals.

THE RIGHT DIET

You can prevent another gallbladder attack by avoiding the rich, high-fat foods that most likely caused the revolt. Studies show that eating a vegetarian diet is the best defense against gallbladder trouble. If this isn't for you, follow these dietary habits.

- Eat six to nine servings or fruits and vegetables a day.
- Focus on fruits and vegetables containing mucilaginous fiber, such as oat bran, pectin (apples and pears), and guar gum.
- Drink eight 8-ounce glasses of water a day. This will help maintain the proper water content of bile.
- Avoid eggs, the number one food most likely to induce a gallbladder attack. Other foods include onions, nuts, corn, coffee, and milk.

PAY ATTENTION TO PREVENTION

To prevent gallstones and gallbladder disease, you should treat your body with the respect it deserves. In addition to following the dietary advice above, you should also do the following.

- Exercise regularly.
- Avoid smoking or spending time around people who do.
- Maintain your ideal weight.
- Avoid crash diets and rapid weight-loss programs, which can cause gallstones.

WHEN TO CALL THE DOCTOR

A gallbladder that's in trouble usually produces pain severe enough to make a trip to the emergency room a no-brainer. This, however, is usually preceded with symptoms that warn you of a pending attack.

Most people with gallstones and gallbladder disease experience the classic symptoms of digestive distress—bloating, gas, and nausea—especially after eating a fatty meal. If you experience these warning signs, contact your doctor.

GASTRITIS

There is one word particularly well suited to stand in as a synonym for gastritis: misery.

Gastritis means several hours, at best, of almost constant vomiting or diarrhea—and most likely both—as a result of a bodily assault from an unfriendly invader. It could have come from something you ate (food poisoning) or from a bug going around school or the office. Sometimes it is accompanied by flulike symptoms, such as chills and fever, and stomach cramping. Whatever the cause, it's got you good and all you care about at the moment is stopping the agony.

Don't do it! As lousy as you feel, you want to let nature take its course. The vomiting and diarrhea are your body's way of ridding your system of the poisonlike offender. At best you'll feel better in 24 hours; at worst, it can last a few days.

The only real threat from gastritis is dehydration and the loss of electrolytes and minerals, which can have serious, even life-threatening, consequences. Here's what to do.

NATURE'S HELPERS

Water. Keep a glass of water by your side and keep sipping it, even if it makes you vomit. If you do vomit, you'll still need to keep drinking the water. Sipping slowly, however, should help prevent it from coming back up.

Gatorade. Any sports drink, such as Gatorade, will help restore electrolytes and minerals quicker than water. If there's none around the house, put a pinch of salt in a glass of water.

Lemon. If you're pretty certain that your current condition was caused by something you ate, squeeze a wedge of lemon juice into your water. Lemon helps in two ways: It increases the acidity in your stomach, making an inhospitable environment for bacteria, and it helps flush out any toxins that might be holing up in your liver.

Miso. Miso, a fermented paste popular in Japanese cuisine, contains enzymes that can help calm your churning stomach. Drink some miso soup when your troubles start to abate. It's a tasty and healthful way to reintroduce your digestive system to food.

WHEN TO CALL THE DOCTOR

Vomiting and diarrhea can cause dehydration very quickly in babies, young children, and the elderly. Don't attempt to wait it out. Call your doctor right away. You should also call the doctor if you have a fever that's over 100 degrees or you see blood when you purge.

GLAUCOMA

Glaucoma is a serious eye disease and one of the leading causes of blindness. It is characterized by increased pressure within the eye, called intraocular pressure, caused by a buildup of fluid in the anterior chamber of the eye.

In a healthy eye, fluid is produced and drained at equal speed. If fluid doesn't drain properly, it builds up and puts pressure on the retina, lens, and optic nerve. If the pressure is severe enough, it can damage or even destroy the retina and optic nerve.

Glaucoma usually progresses slowly. At first, the buildup of fluid produces no symptoms. But as pressure builds, peripheral vision narrows. Halos can appear in your range of sight and you can have trouble adapting to the dark. It can also produce mild headaches.

Although rare, glaucoma can come on suddenly and is considered a medical emergency. Acute glaucoma usually occurs in one eye only and is accompanied by severe throbbing pain in the affected eye, blurred vision, a moderately dilated pupil, nausea, and vomiting.

Glaucoma needs to be closely monitored by an ophthalmologist. Treatment of both types of glaucoma involves reducing the amount of pressure in the eye and improving the metabolism of collagen in the eye. Treatment includes drugs and/or surgery. In addition to professional care, here are some natural ways to help protect your vision.

Magnesium. This important mineral helps relax blood vessel walls and improve blood flow to the eye. One study found daily supplementation helped improve the visual field of people with glaucoma.

Recommended dosage: Take 250 milligrams twice a day.

Vitamin C. This antioxidant is important because it helps reduce intraocular pressure.

Recommended dosage: Take 1,000 milligrams up to four times a day.

Berries. Anthocyanoside, the pigment found in the skin of blueberries, bilberries, huckleberries, and cranberries, helps increase the activity of vitamin C. Eat them to your heart's desire or take capsules.

Recommended dosage: Take 240 to 480 milligrams of standardized 25-percent anthocyanosides a day.

Rutin. Naturopathic physicians treat glaucoma with rutin, a bioflavonoid found in the wild pansy that helps lower intraocular pressure.

Recommended dosage: 20 milligrams three times a day.

PAY ATTENTION TO PREVENTION

Glaucoma is not totally preventable. If you have a family history of glaucoma, you can help reduce your risk of developing the disease by eating a diet high in vitamin C and omega-3 fatty acids (salmon, mackerel, herring, and other cold-water fish). Avoid corticosteroid drugs such as prednisone, which weaken collagen structures, including those in the eye.

WHEN TO CALL THE DOCTOR

Acute glaucoma is a medical emergency that needs immediate treatment. If you have any of the signs of acute glaucoma described above call your doctor or ophthalmologist now. If not treated within 12 to 48 hours, acute glaucoma can result in permanent blindness.

GOUT

If you want to see a grown man cry, find one with a big toe swollen by gout.

Gout, a form of arthritis, is the excessive buildup of uric acid crystals that results from an excess of rich food and drink. It causes excruciating pain.

Back in the seventeenth century, having gout was a sign of wealth because only the rich could afford to partake in the good drink and rich food associated with the condition.

How times change. Nowadays no income level is required to join the gout club. But it does favor men: over 95 percent of people who know gout are overweight males over the age of 30. It also favors a family membership—you can inherit a tendency to get gout.

PURINE: A GOUT CHOW

Uric acid is manufactured from purine, a substance most abundant in organ meats (liver, kidneys, sweetbreads), gravy, and beer. Your body also produces uric acid. So, when you get too much through eating high-purine foods, the acid forms into tiny crystals called tophi. These excess crystals have to go somewhere. Often, like a lump of sugar plunked in a cup of coffee, they go straight to the bottom—and settle in the first joint of the big toe. Less commonly they settle in the ankle, heel, or instep.

Gout is unpredictable and can appear without warning. When it strikes, the five-alarm pain leaves no doubt as to what you've got. Anyone who has experienced gout once say they never want to do so again. This is why many men opt for a lifetime on the daily drug allopurinol, which is very effective at avoiding an attack. If you want to avoid the drug, or simply want extra insurance, these are your choices.

OUT WITH GOUT

Celery. Celery extract helps remove uric acid from the body and may be as effective as allopurinol at avoiding gout. Eat several stalks of celery a day and take an herbal supplement.

Recommended dosage: 2 to 4 tablets of celery seed extract once a day.

Cherry. There is abundant anecdotal evidence that eating cherries every day will prevent a gout attack. That's any kind of cherries—fresh, canned, even maraschino. Or drink black cherry juice, which you can find as a concentrate in health food stores.

Recommended dosage: Mix 1 tablespoon black cherry concentrate in an 8-ounce glass of water and drink once a day.

Devil's Claw. Studies show that this natural anti-inflammatory herb is effective at reducing gout pain and dissolving uric acid crystals.

Recommended dosage: Take 1,500 to 2,500 milligrams a day.

Stinging nettle. Doctors in Europe use the leaf of stinging nettle to reduce the uric acid buildup associated with gout.

Recommended dosage: Take two 600-milligram capsules twice a day.

Chiso. The Japanese have long used this mint-flavored weed to relieve gout. Add it to boiling water and steep to make a tea, or do like the Japanese and put it in a sushi roll.

PAY ATTENTION TO PREVENTION

The best way to avoid gout is to avoid foods high in purines. These are the most egregious offenders.

- Anchovies
- Beer
- Game
- Gravy
- Herring
- Liver
- Kidneys
- Mackerel
- Meat extracts
- Sardines
- Scallops
- Sweetbreads

In addition, some recommendations are as follows.

- Limit alcohol consumption to 3 drinks a week.
- Drink 8 glasses of water a day to dilute and eliminate uric acid through urine.

- Choose lean cuts of meat over fatty meats.
- Eat lentils, peas, beans, asparagus, cauliflower, spinach, and mushrooms in small amounts, as these foods also contain purines.

GUM DISEASE

Your smile is the mirror to your health—and it has nothing to do with the brightening strips you slide on your teeth at night. Oral health is about wearing a smile free of what you can't see—bacteria that hide behind tartar and burrow into gums.

Your mouth is continually exposed to billions of bacteria and microscopic organisms that influence the health of your teeth and gums. As you chew, the acids in sugars and starches release a sticky film of bacteria that clings to the teeth. If the bacteria are not removed through diligent brushing, it hardens into plaque and produces toxins that irritate the gums. If left unattended, however, the irritation causes gums to swell, turn red, and easily bleed—all signs of infection known as gingivitis. These toxins eventually burrow into the gums and form pockets, making more room for bacterial deposits. This digression forewarns periodontal disease, a serious condition that can destroy the soft tissue that supports the teeth and can ultimately lead to losing some or all of your teeth.

While inadequate dental hygiene is the major cause of periodontal disease, other contributing factors include habitual clenching and grinding of the teeth, a high-sugar diet, and the use of tobacco, drugs, and alcohol. Heredity, hormonal imbalances, and stress are other possible factors.

TOOTHPASTE TOO TASTY?

The key to exceptional oral health is to clean your teeth morning, night, and after meals with a toothpaste containing the fastest and most effective bacteria-destroying natural and active ingredients. And you won't necessarily find them in commercial toothpastes.

Commercial toothpastes tend to focus more on artificial sweeteners, for the best taste, and whiteners, for the best shine, rather than fast-killing natural bacterial agents. This is why dentists often say that you're better off brushing your teeth with baking soda than commercial toothpaste.

You can find a variety of natural toothpaste in health food stores and through Internet catalogs. Look for toothpaste containing these ingredients.

GUM-FRIENDLY NUTRIENTS

Coenzyme Q10. This naturally occurring compound integral to the health of body cells acts as an antioxidant and is well known for its ability to help decrease the depth of periodontal pockets and heal gums in people with periodontitis. In one experiment, it was so effective that researchers had difficultly locating the disease in the gums of those infected. If you already have gum disease, consider taking a supplement in addition to using a toothpaste containing CoQ10.

Recommended Dosage: 50 to 150 milligrams a day.

Pomegranate. Scientists in Brazil found that pomegranate extract has the ability to kill bacteria that resist regular brushing and lead to the formation of hard-to-remove tartar.

Squalene. An extract of shark liver oil, squalene has potent antioxidant properties.

Tea Tree. The volatile oil in tea tree is important to maintaining healthy tissue. If you have sore gums, put two or three drops in a shot glass of warm water and swish it around your mouth.

Lactoferrin. This protein, which belongs to the iron family, is a well-known immune system booster effective at controlling infectious assault, trauma, and injury.

Sanguinarine. The active ingredient in bloodroot has been proven effective against oral bacteria.

Peppermint. You can't count on the "peppermint" found in commercial toothpaste to promote dental health, but real peppermint does help fight bacteria and tooth decay. Chew on fresh mint leaves or enjoy it as a tea.

PAY ATTENTION TO PREVENTION

Good dental health requires diligent brushing and flossing. You can also save your teeth by eating a diet that is rich in antioxidant vegetables and fruits and low in sugar and sweets.

Some dentists believe an electric toothbrush stimulates the gums in addition to cleaning the teeth, so consider using one if your dentist recommends it.

Avoid mouthwashes with alcohol, which can dry out and irritate sensitive gums. And, of course, have your teeth professionally cleaned twice a year, or more often if you already have periodontal disease.

WHEN TO CALL THE DOCTOR

If your gums are tender and sore and bleed when you brush you teeth, discuss it with your dentist at the first opportunity. These are signs of possible gum disease.

HANGOVER

It's a beautiful morning—but not for you. Somehow, your happy hour the night before turned into a few too many. And now you're paying your dues.

Alcohol does more than deplete you of inhibitions. It depletes you of fluid and electrolytes. Putting water and nutrients back in your body will help you feel better but they are not a cure. The only real cure for a hangover is time. These remedies should help you get through the in-between time.

HANGOVER HELPERS

Fructose. The sugar in fruit can accelerate the metabolism of alcohol by 25 percent, according to Asian researchers. Perhaps this is why a Bloody Mary, a concoction of vodka and tomato, is such a common day-after remedy. It's better to take the juice straight, however. Also try orange or grapefruit juice.

Honey. It's another form of fructose. Mix a few tablespoons in a glass of water and drink.

Ginseng. Both American and Asian ginseng are age-old remedies for a hangover.

Recommended dosage: 200–400 milligrams.

Angostura. Bitter herbs, such as angostura, help relieve a hangover, according to Chinese herbalists. Put several drops in a cup of hot water and drink it as a morning-after tea.

Cinchona. This is another bitter herb like angostura. Mix in a glass of water and drink.

Nux vomica. This homeopathic remedy is considered an antidote for hangover.

Recommended dosage: Dissolve 3 pellets of 30C nux vomica on the tongue every four hours.

PAY ATTENTION TO PREVENTION

Let's bypass the lecture on the evils of alcohol. If you're going to drink, do so sensibly.

Drink slowly. The body of a 150-pound man burns an

average of one ounce of alcohol an hour. Keep this, and *your own size and tolerance*, in mind. The more slowly you drink, the less alcohol will reach your brain.

Eat. Never drink on an empty stomach. Food slows the absorption of alcohol.

Avoid the bubbly. This doesn't just mean champagne. Anything with bubbles put alcohol into the bloodstream quicker.

Think light. The rule of thumb: The darker the alcohol, the harder it will be on you the next day.

HEADACHES AND MIGRAINES

Headaches are more common than the common cold. Estimates indicate that 90 percent of people *the world over* are familiar with headache pain. That's a lot of pain!

Headaches come in three varieties: tension headaches, migraines, and cluster headaches.

Tension headaches, by far, are the most common. Despite what the name implies, however, they are not always caused by emotional tension. Almost anything can cause a tension headache—working too long and too hard, muscle strain, driving in bright sunlight, poor posture, even eating certain foods. Whatever the trigger, it causes the muscles in the face or neck to contract, creating throbbing and pain around the eyes, temples, or ears.

A migraine, however, is something else altogether. Migraines are intense, throbbing pain that result from vessels swelling in the head. They can cause nausea, vomiting, blurred vision, and sensitivity to light. For some people, they are debilitating. What brings on a migraine differs from person to person but common triggers include wine, chocolate, cheese, and hormonal changes. The later is the reason why three times as many women are plagued with migraines than men.

Cluster headaches are the most rare and are considered the most painful. The pain, described as "stabbing," centers around one side of the head. Thankfully, they are short lived, lasting for a few minutes to no more than a few hours.

Some 40 million people in the United States suffer from chronic headaches that drive them to the doctor, seeking relief. While there are plenty of prescription and over-the-counter medications that will relieve a headache, there are also some tried-and-true natural remedies that are just as effective. Keep in mind, however, that what works for one person doesn't necessarily help another—and this includes pharmaceutical medications.

NATURAL PAIN RELIEVERS

Feverfew. Clinical studies have found that feverfew is powerful at preventing and reducing the frequency of migraine headaches. Feverfew works by inhibiting substances that dilate blood vessels. Dosages vary depending on the potency of the product; take according to package directions. Or take it as a fluid extract.

Recommended dosage: Take one-fourth to one half teaspoon of fluid extract three times daily.

5-HTP. 5-hydroxytryptophan is shown to be effective against both tension and migraine headaches. It helps boost serotonin, which helps keeps blood circulating in the brain.

Recommended dosage: Take 50 to 100 milligrams three times a day.

Magnesium. Headache-prone people tend to have low levels of magnesium in the blood. There is also evidence showing that taking magnesium can relieve both migraine and tension headaches.

Recommended dosage: Take 250 to 400 milligrams three times daily.

Ginger. This is a well-known cure for migraines in Asia. Try it in a tea or take as a capsule.

Recommended dosage: Take 500 milligrams in capsules a day.

Peppermint. The volatile oil in peppermint can help relieve spasms and tension in the body. Mix a few drops in a tablespoon of nonscented lotion or olive oil and rub it against your temples.

Homeopathic headache formula. Look for one with a combination formula and take as directed.

PAY ATTENTION TO PREVENTION

If you get frequent headaches you may benefit from any variety of stress-relief methods, including meditation, progressive relation, and yoga. You should also examine your diet, especially if you get migraine headaches.

WHEN TO CALL THE DOCTOR

Most headaches amount to little more than an occasional inconvenience. In rare cases, however, headaches are warning signs of a serious health problem. Make sure to discuss this with your doctor.

You should also call the doctor if you develop a headache following a head injury, sneeze or sudden cough, or if a headache is accompanied by fever, stiff neck, lethargy, or vomiting.

HEARTBURN

Heartburn is the painful price you pay for having a love affair with food that doesn't love you back.

When you eat the wrong food with abandon, or you eat

something your stomach just can't tolerate, it gets every tom, dick, and enzyme from one end of the chow line to the other in a digestive uproar. There are lots of foods a persnickety stomach can't take in big doses—coffee, chocolate, and spices, just to name a few—but there is one family in particular that it finds simply too unsavory: *The Acids.*

Acids don't start raising a ruckus until they get through a flap of muscular tissue called the lower esophageal sphincter (LES). The LES acts like a trap door—a safeguard for the continued one-way passage through the digestive tract. But the stomach doesn't always see it this way. When acid gets to be too much, the stomach rebels and forces it back through the trap door. Suddenly going the wrong way on a one-way route, it seeks refuge in the first safe haven it can find—the middle of your breastbone, where it painfully lets you know that the road to love does not always run smooth.

FIGHTING BACK

For some people with discriminating stomachs, it doesn't matter how hard you try—such as putting the jalapeño-stuffed tomato sauce on a bed of brown rice, for example—you just can't change a hostile acid environment. If giving up the food you love is out of the question, you can try patching things up with these peacemakers.

Ginger. Drink a cup of ginger tea after eating a heartburn-causing meal and likely you won't feel any discomfort at all. Ginger is a powerful stomach soother.

Licorice. A form of licorice called deglycyrrhizinated licorice (DGL) is an antispasmodic that helps reduce the production of stomach acid, thereby decreasing heartburn. Licorice however is not for long-term use, but it's okay to take for an occasional, sudden acid attack.

Recommended dosage: Take one 200- to 300-milligram DGL chewable tablet, no more than three a day.

Carrot juice. The alkalinity in carrots helps reduce acid in the stomach. Drink a glass of juice when you feel the symptoms coming on.

Seeds. Instead of popping an antacid, chew on one or a combination of anise, caraway, or fennel seeds—all herbs that help soothe the stomach.

Kim chi. If you have chronic indigestion, introduce fermented foods into your diet, such as raw cultured vegetables, sauerkraut and kim chi. Fermented foods help promote good digestion.

PAY ATTENTION TO PREVENTION

Heartburn is one of those ailments that is much easier to avoid than cure. To minimize your risk of developing heartburn, don't aggravate your stomach. For one, don't overeat. If you can't cut back (or you don't need to), increase the number of meals you eat each day and decrease the portions. Just make sure you don't start eating more. Also, ask yourself, *"Is this going to be worth it?"* before reaching for any of these notorious heart burners.

- Beer
- Caffeinated beverages, such as coffee, tea, and colas
- Carbonated beverages
- Chocolate
- Citrus
- Fatty food
- Fried food
- Tomatoes

WHEN TO CALL THE DOCTOR

As you probably know, more people with heartburn go to the hospital with symptoms of a heart attack than people who are actually having a heart attack. However, this doesn't mean you should hesitate about heading to the hospital, even if you are the least bit unsure. Embarrassment is nothing compared to the consequences of getting too late to the hospital with a heart attack.

Also, get to the emergency room if chest pain is accompanied by shortness of breath; pain in the neck, back, or down your right arm; and/or dizziness.

Occasional heartburn isn't serious but recurrent and frequent bouts could be a sign of something awry somewhere in the body, such as an ulcer or gastroesophageal reflux disease (GERD). Contact your doctor if you experience heartburn three or four times a week for several weeks.

HEART DISEASE

Cancer is the disease people fear the most, but heart disease is what kills the most people. In fact, heart disease is the number-one killer of both men and women worldwide.

Heart disease isn't something that comes on suddenly like the cold or the flu. It develops slowly, manifesting itself over years and starting, in some instances, as early as childhood. It can be so sneaky, in fact, that 64 percent of women and 50 percent of men who die suddenly from a heart attack had no known symptoms.

This is why it is so important to know your heart disease risk. Even if you are genetically prone to heart disease, it does not mean that getting it is inevitable. Heart disease is preventable—mostly by the way you choose to live your life.

These are the leading risk factors contributing to heart disease.

- Smoking
- A diet high in saturated fat
- Lack of exercise
- High blood pressure
- High cholesterol, especially high LDL cholesterol
- Elevated triglycerides
- Overweight, especially excess weight around the waist
- Diabetes
- Prediabetes
- Elevated levels of C-reactive protein (CRP), a sign of low-grade inflammation in the bloodstream ·

The more risk factors you have, the greater your risk of developing heart disease.

ANATOMY OF AN ARTERY

Cardiovascular disease is an umbrella term for "hardening of the arteries," the accumulation of plaque on artery walls. Plaque is caused by fatty deposits in the bloodstream that cling to artery walls and harden. As plaque accumulates, arteries narrow and restrict the flow of oxygen-carrying blood to the heart.

The heart muscle is so efficient at extracting oxygen from the blood that an artery can be 70 to 90 percent blocked before any symptoms, such as pain or tightness in the chest, appear. When one or more of the coronary arteries become completely blocked, the result is a heart attack. When the blockage occurs in an artery leading to the brain, the result is a stroke. Unfortunately for some, a heart attack or stroke is the first warning sign that something is wrong.

Whether you've had a heart attack or want to avoid one, it is never too late to take action to protect your heart.

EAT TO YOUR HEART'S CONTENT

Forget what you shouldn't eat. Concentrate on what you *can* eat. There are many delicious heart-healthy foods to keep your taste buds content. Add these foods to your diet in place of artery-clogging fat and cholesterol.

Mediterranean foods. Numerous studies show that populations that adhere to a traditional Mediterranean diet have the lowest rate of heart disease in the world. A traditional Mediterranean diet has these characteristics.

- Low in saturated fat (meaning meat and butter)
- High in antioxidant-rich fruits and vegetables
- High in cholesterol-controlling legumes and whole grains
- Abundant in fish (a minimum of three to five times a week) containing heart-protecting omega-3 fatty acids

Extra virgin olive oil. The Mediterranean diet is low in saturated fat, but it is not a low-fat diet. Scientists believe that the lion's share of heart protection in the Mediterranean diet comes from olive oil, the richest source of mono-unsaturated fat. Mono fat has the unique ability to lower bad LDL cholesterol and raise good HDL cholesterol. Use olive oil in your recipes in place of butter. Other oils that are good sources of monos are canola, almond, and avocado.

Red wine. Mediterraneans are also noted for their large consumption of wine. Scientists have identified more than 500 active substances in wine that they believe work synergistically to alter blood chemistry in ways that help lower cholesterol and prevent other processes that lead to hardening of the arteries. Two substances in particular, the polyphenols resveratrol and saponins, are most abundant in wine. Red wine has ten times more polyphenols than white wine.

Recommended serving: Women should drink one 5-ounce glass of wine and men two 5-ounce glasses of wine a day.

Chocolate. Like wine, chocolate is loaded with special nutrients that do the heart good. Specifically, chocolate contains a class of polyphenols called flavanols. Dark chocolate contains more flavanols than any other food.

Recommended serving: Eat up to 2-ounces of dark chocolate a day.

Tomatoes. A seven-year study of 40,000 middle-aged and older women found that those who consumed seven to ten servings a week of tomato-based products had a 29 percent lower risk of heart disease than women who ate one and a half servings a week. Tomatoes are rich in vitamin A, vitamin C, folate, potassium, and lycopene—nutrients that each protect the heart in special ways.

Blueberries. These tiny berries are not only brimming with antioxidants, but they contain a compound called ellagic acid, which helps reduce inflammation in the body that puts the heart at risk.

Broccoli. This rich source of flavonols stands out as a significant contributor in helping reduce the risk of heart disease. It also contains heart-protecting vitamin C, folate, and potassium.

Pomegranate juice. A rich source of antioxidants, drinking pomegranate juice has been shown to lower bad LDL cholesterol and improve blood flow to the heart.

HEART-SMART SUPPLEMENTS

If you have heart disease or take any medication to control risk factors such as high cholesterol and high blood pressure, check with your doctor before taking any supplements.

Fish oil. There are numerous studies that show that fish oil has a positive influence on heart health. If you can't stand the thought of eating fish several times a week, then opt for a fish oil capsule.

Recommended dosage: Take a fish oil product containing 480 milligrams of EPA and 360 milligrams of DHA a day.

Folate and B12. High levels of homocysteine in the blood are associated with high levels of C-reactive protein. Studies have found that the B vitamin folate and vitamin B12 work in tandem to help reduce homocysteine.

Recommended dosage: Take 800 micrograms of folate and 800 micrograms of vitamin B12 daily.

Hawthorn. Research shows that this well-known heart herb helps prevent a heart attack. It improves blood circulation and increases the heart's ability to deal with reduced oxygen intake.

Recommended dosage: Take 450 to 900 milligrams a day.

Antioxidants. Take an antioxidant formula containing beta-carotene, vitamin C, vitamin E, and selenium.

LIVE TO LIVE WELL

Eating right is only part of the formula that prevents heart disease or makes living with heart disease a lot less risky. Incorporate these lifestyle factors into your life.

Exercise. Most doctors agree that an active lifestyle that includes exercise is even more important than diet when it comes to protecting your heart. Exercise is considered walking at least 30 minutes a day at least five days a week.

Be slim. The majority of people who have a heart attack are overweight.

Avoid trans fats. Trans fats are double trouble. They are bad because, like saturated fat, they lead to a buildup of fat on artery walls. Even worse, they increase levels of bad LDL cholesterol and lower levels of good HDL cholesterol.

Avoid stress. There is a correlation between high stress and high risk for heart attack.

Get social. Research shows that people who are socially active and have a network of friends are less likely to have a heart attack than people who are socially isolated.

WHEN TO CALL THE DOCTOR

Unrelenting tightness and pain in the chest is a common symptom of a heart attack but it is not always the most severe or prominent symptom in women.

Women can experience more flulike symptoms such as back and neck pain, pressure in the upper abdomen, and unrelenting fatigue.

If you are experiencing chest pain, don't try to second-guess what it might be. Get medical help right away.

HEMORRHOIDS

The ancient Greek physician Hippocrates thought he had a sure-fire cure for hemorrhoids—burning them away with a red-hot iron.

Thank heaven—and savvy herbalists, among others—that there is no need today to go to such drastic measures. If there were a lot of people would be running in the opposite direction because hemorrhoids is one of the most common conditions among modern man and woman. An estimated one out of three people suffer from these uncomfortable, itchy, and sometimes bleeding bubbles on the inner flesh of the butt.

BLEEDING VEIN

Hemorrhoids are masses of swollen veins in the lower rectum or anus. The condition develops from increased pressure in the veins in the lower rectum as a result of chronic constipation and straining to have a bowel movement. Other common causes of hemorrhoids include diarrhea, obesity, and spending too much time sitting on the toilet. They are also common among pregnant women when the fetus starts putting increased pressure on the rectal area.

Hemorrhoids can pop up both inside the rectum and outside. The most common signs of internal hemorrhoids are traces of bright red blood on toilet paper and in the toilet bowl. Burning, discomfort, and itching may result if external hemorrhoids become irritated.

Hemorrhoids are harmless, but they are also a real pain in the you-know-what. Here is what you can do to get some relief.

Butcher's Broom. This herb with the funny name has a long history as an herbal remedy for hemorrhoids. Its healing action comes from chemicals called ruscogenins, which have the ability to help veins constrict. Make a tincture by mixing it with alcohol or take a supplement.

Recommended dosage: 200 milligrams a day.

Horse chestnut. The bark of this tree contains several agents that help dissolve hemorrhoids. You can take it orally but the herb has a tendency to cause constipation, which can make hemorrhoids worse. Instead, use the herb to make a strong tea and apply it as you would a lotion.

Witch hazel. This is a soothing, cool astringent that is the active ingredient in some over-the-counter hemorrhoid ointments. Lightly soak a cotton pad with witch hazel and tuck it around your hemorrhoids.

Bioflavonoids. Several types of bioflavonoids have been found effective at reducing hemorrhoids.

Recommended dosage: Take 1,000 milligrams of bioflavonoids twice a day.

PAY ATTENTION TO PREVENTION

You can prevent hemmorhoids the same way you prevent constipation. See page 95 for safe and effective remedies.

WHEN TO CALL THE DOCTOR

Never assume rectal bleeding is from hemorrhoids. See your doctor to rule out cancer or other disease.

HYPERTENSION

High blood pressure is a sneaky stalker. You can't see it. You can't feel it. You can't even figure out why it is targeting *you*. Right now, some 50 million Americans are being stalked by high blood pressure and half of them don't even know it—yet.

High blood pressure is an exasperating condition to treat. It leaves no clues that it is sneaking up on you. It can be fine one minute and way too high 15 minutes later. This is why high blood pressure, or hypertension, is called the silent killer and is one of the most seriously taken threats to health. In fact, it is the most accurate predictor of future cardiovascular disease in people over age 65.

WHAT'S NORMAL, WHAT ISN'T

Simply put, hypertension means that the force of blood against artery walls is stronger than normal. The systolic reading (the top number on a blood pressure reading) measures the pressure of blood against artery walls when the heart has just finished contracting, or pumping, blood. The diastolic reading (the bottom number) is the pressure of blood against artery walls between beats when the heart is relaxed and filling with blood.

Ninety percent of the time, doctors aren't sure what causes high blood pressure, but they do know that it wears and tears at the arteries of the heart, setting you up for a heart attack or stroke.

Blood pressure has a tendency to rise with weight gain and is more prevalent in blacks than in whites. It is more dangerous for women than it is for men because older women are more prone to a stroke.

Ideally, your blood pressure should be less than 120/80 mm Hg. High blood pressure is considered to be greater than 140/90 mm Hg. Studies show, however, that a "high normal reading"—systolic between 130 and 139 and diastolic between 80 and 89—can be just as risky.

Fortunately, losing weight and making other positive life-style changes can control most cases of high blood pressure.

BRING THE PRESSURE DOWN

Coenzyme Q10. This essential component of the mitrochondria, the energy-producing unit of a cell, is involved in chemical processes that keep blood pressure stable. CoQ10 levels decline with age.

Recommended dosage: Take 100 milligrams twice a day.

Garlic. Allicin is the substance that makes garlic heart healthy and that includes helping to keep blood pressure down. Garlic has been shown to lower systolic pressure by an impressive 20 to 30 mm Hg and diastolic by 10 to 20 mm Hg. Use garlic in your cooking on a daily basis. You can also take a garlic supplement.

Recommended dosage: Take 600 milligrams twice a day.

Hawthorn. This herb from the hawthorn tree gets rave reviews from natural healers for its ability to help lower blood pressure.

Recommended dosage: Take two 500-milligram capsules three times a day.

Potassium. Low levels of potassium, especially when combined with high levels of sodium, increase fluid retention and inhibit the body's blood-pressure-regulating system. If you are taking diuretics or high-blood-pressure medication, you may need a daily potassium supplement. Your doctor should determine this.

Magnesium and Calcium. Low levels of these minerals have also been associated with high blood pressure. Ask your doctor to check your blood levels of these nutrients. Take supplements under the direction of your doctor.

Vitamin C. One study found that taking as little as 250 milligrams of vitamin C daily slashed the risk of high blood pressure by almost half.

Recommended dosage: Take 1,500 milligrams of vitamin C daily.

Saffron. This expensive herb, which is used widely in Spanish cuisine, contains the blood pressure-lowering substance crocetin. Some scientist speculates that Spain's low incidence of heart disease is due to consumption of crocetin-rich saffron.

Reishi. Chinese physician use this oriental mushroom to help control blood pressure. You can buy it in capsule form.

Recommended dosage: Take up to 4,000 milligrams a day.

PAY ATTENTION TO PREVENTION

Everyone should be intimate with his or her blood pressure. In addition to having it checked at the doctor's office, you can check it yourself with a blood pressure monitor. Make sure to follow the instructions carefully.

Even people who lead healthy lives can end up with high blood pressure. Nevertheless, these lifestyle practices can help keep your blood pressure where it belongs.

Don't smoke, and avoid being around people who do. Nicotine constricts the arteries and elevates blood pressure. A person with uncontrolled hypertension who smokes is five times more likely to have a heart attack and sixteen times more likely to have a stroke than a non-smoker.

Lose weight, if necessary. Obesity is a leading cause of high blood pressure. An analysis of five studies involving weight loss and hypertension found that, on average, losing 20 pounds resulted in a decline of 6.3 mm Hg in systolic and 3.1 mm Hg in diastolic pressure.

Monitor your use of over-the-counter medicines. Avoid using antihistamines, decongestants, cold remedies, and appetite suppressants, unless recommended by a doctor.

Manage your daily stress. Stress can temporarily elevate blood pressure. Relaxation techniques such as biofeedback, meditation, yoga, progressive muscle relaxation, and hypnosis have been shown to help lower blood pressure.

Restrict alcohol consumption. While research shows cardiovascular benefits from modest drinking, just one drink a day can raise blood pressure levels in some people.

WHEN TO CALL THE DOCTOR

If you have high blood pressure and experience any of the following symptoms, call your doctor. They are an indication that your blood pressure is not being adequately controlled.

- Frequent headaches
- Shortness of breath
- Fatigue
- Heart palpitations
- Nose bleeds
- Flushing in the face

INCONTINENCE

Oops—didn't mean to do that.

Loss of bladder control, or urinary incontinence, is a distressing condition for obvious reasons. It's also one of those conditions people don't like to talk about. But more than 10 million people have it, including at least 10 to 20 percent of all older adults.

Before age 65, incontinence affects three to five times more women than men. Women who have had children experience more problems because pregnancy places intense pressure on the bladder and muscles of the pelvic floor; in addition, labor and delivery can tear the muscles and surrounding tissues, sometimes leaving them less resilient than before. About 40 percent of women experience some incontinence during pregnancy, and 10 percent continue to have problems afterward. At menopause, the decrease in estrogen can weaken the pelvic floor muscles and thin the lining of the urethra, loosening the seal at the neck of the bladder.

Men experience less incontinence, in part because they have longer urethras (10 inches, versus about 2 inches for women). The prostate gland also helps support a man's urethra, helping to prevent leakage. An enlarged prostate, however, can put pressure on the bladder, so that after age 65 men and women have an almost equal chance of becoming incontinent.

FIVE DIFFERENT VARIETIES

There are five basic types of chronic incontinence. Stress incontinence is a condition in which you experience dribbles of urine loss when you exercise, cough, laugh, sneeze, or move in other ways that put pressure on the bladder. Most cases of stress incontinence are associated with weak muscles in the pelvic floor, though in severe cases there may be nerve damage or tears in the sphincter muscles.

Urge incontinence usually involves the loss of a larger amount of urine with little warning. It occurs when the need to urinate comes on so quickly that there isn't enough time to make it to the toilet. Urge incontinence can be caused by stroke, Parkinson's disease, kidney or bladder stones, or bladder infection.

Overflow incontinence involves urination with no warning or sensation. In such cases urine spills unexpectedly when you shift position or stand up. You may feel the need to urinate again a few minutes later but are unable to empty the bladder completely. Pelvic or bladder surgery, diabetes, and an enlarged prostate can cause overflow incontinence. People with overflow incontinence have a high risk of bladder infection.

Reflex incontinence involves involuntary, spontaneous urination—no warnings, no urges, no rush to the bathroom. This lack of bladder control is usually caused by spinal cord injury, diabetes, multiple sclerosis, and other serious medical conditions.

Functional incontinence strikes people who have normal bladder control and warnings but cannot reach the bathroom fast enough due to physical limitations.

Temporary incontinence can be caused by the use of diuretics and other medications.

In many cases, incontinence will go away along with the

condition that is causing it. But this doesn't mean that others need to accept it as a fact of life. There are ways to control it.

BLADDER CONTROL

Kegels. This simple exercise, named after the Arnold Kegel, M.D., the doctor who invented it, is very effective at toning and strengthening the pelvic floor, thus controlling incontinence:

- Locate the appropriate muscles by repeatedly stopping your urine in midstream. The muscles you squeeze around your urethra and anus to stop the urine are the muscles you want to work.
- Practice squeezing then releasing these muscles several times each day when you urinate. Once you are familiar with them, practice squeezing them when you are not urinating.
- During each exercise contraction, hold the squeeze for three seconds, then relax for three seconds. Repeat this 10 to 15 times per session, three or four sessions a day.

Double void. Another way to help control incontinence is through double voiding. Empty your bladder, then relax a minute and try again. You might also try urinating, then standing up for a minute, sitting down and leaning forward, then trying again.

Lose weight. Extra pounds can also cause the pelvic floor to sag, giving you yet another good reason to shed the extra weight.

Don't smoke. Nicotine in cigarettes irritates the bladder and a smoker's cough can cause problems with stress incontinence.

HERBAL HELPERS

Horsetail. Also called bottlebrush, this abrasive plant contains silica, which helps support the regeneration of connective tissue. Drink it as a tea in combination with doing Kegels.

Black cohosh has mild estrogen effects, meaning it acts like the female hormone estrogen, which can help strengthen the muscles in the pelvic floor. Commercial products are available; follow package directions.

Kava kava. This herb can help if you have an irritable bladder. Don't take it before going to bed, however, as it can increase urination.

Recommended dosage: Take 30 drops of tincture with water three times a day.

WHEN TO CALL THE DOCTOR

If you experience incontinence, talk to your doctor about the problem. More than half of all people with incontinence fail to seek help, though experts estimate that more than 80 percent can overcome the problem.

INFERTILITY

Infertility is an incessant roller-coaster ride of promise and possibility, followed by disappointment and despair.

Medically, a couple is considered infertile after having unprotected sexual intercourse regularly during ovulation for a year or more. A woman is also considered infertile if she has a problem carrying a pregnancy to full term. However, only a couple that has tried unsuccessfully to have a child understands that infertility involves much more than this—it can also be an emotionally devastating experience.

Responsibility for infertility is evenly divided between

men and women: about 40 percent of cases can be traced to a problem with the woman, 40 percent can be traced to the man, and 20 percent involve both.

COMMON CAUSES

The most common causes of infertility among women are a failure to ovulate (which is often caused by a hormone imbalance) and a blocked passage of the egg from the ovary to the uterus (which is often associated with endometriosis, infection, or growths).

Other causes include sexually transmitted diseases, pelvic inflammatory disease, smoking, excessive consumption of caffeine, being overweight or underweight, and age (fertility decreases after age 35).

Occasionally an iron deficiency causes infertility in women. Before taking an iron supplement, however, an iron deficiency should be verified by a physician.

Among men the problem may be a low sperm count, low motility (sperm movement is impaired), malformed sperm, or blocked sperm ducts. Wearing tight underwear or pants may temporarily raise the temperature of the testicles, which reduces sperm production.

In both men and women fertility can be adversely affected by depression, anxiety, or exposure to radiation, pesticides, or other environmental poisons.

NATURE'S HELPERS FOR WOMEN

Chasteberry. This herb is helpful to women who don't have regular periods and who have ovaries that don't release eggs monthly.

Recommended dosage: Take 175 milligrams each morning until menstruation becomes normal.

Folate. Folate is important to a healthy pregnancy, so it only makes sense to make sure you are getting adequate amounts if you want to get pregnant. Eat plenty of foods containing folate and take a supplement.

Recommended dosage: Take 400 micrograms a day.

NATURE'S HELPERS FOR MEN

L-Arginine. This amino acid helps improve male sperm count. In one study, 74 percent of 178 men showed significant improvements in sperm count and motility after taking arginine.

Recommended dosage: Take 2,000 milligrams twice a day on an empty stomach.

Zinc. Zinc is involved in hormone metabolism, sperm formation, and sperm motility. Studies show that zinc supplements can help improve testosterone levels and sperm count. Zinc supplements can cause a copper deficiency, so you should also take copper.

Recommended dosage: Take 25 milligrams three times daily and 3 to 5 milligrams of copper.

Ginger. According to Asian researchers, ginger helps enhance sperm count and motility.

Recommended dosage: Take 500 milligrams twice a day.

Vitamin B12. This B vitamin has been shown to help improve sperm count.

Recommended dosage: Take 1,500 micrograms a day.

MEN AND WOMEN

Both vitamin C and vitamin E are important to fertility. Vitamin C, in particular, is helpful to sperm activity.

Recommended dosage: Take 500 milligrams of vitamin C twice a day and 400 I.U. of vitamin E once a day.

PAY ATTENTION TO PREVENTION

Several months before you plan to begin trying to conceive, take steps to minimize your consumption of alcohol and medications, including over-the-counter drugs. Men should avoid hot tubs, which can impair sperm production.

WHEN TO CALL THE DOCTOR

If you are having problems conceiving discuss it with your doctor. Your doctor can test your hormone levels and run a few screening tests to see if you have a simple problem that is affecting your fertility. Your doctor may want to refer you to a fertility expert.

INSOMNIA

Insomnia can be a nightmare. You're desperate for sleep, but it seems that the more exhausted you feel, the harder it is to rest.

Up to 30 percent of Americans have insomnia, which refers to any of three sleep disorders.

- Difficulty falling asleep—you're still awake after 45 minutes.
- Early morning awakening—you wake up at 3 or 4 AM and can't get back to sleep.
- Frequent night awakenings—you wake up six or more times a night.

You have insomnia, however, only if you experience these symptoms and they leave you tired and worn down the next day. After all, you are the ultimate judge of how much pillow time your body needs.

CAUSES OF WAKEFULNESS

Approximately ten million people take prescription drugs to help them sleep, while many more take over-the-counter sleep aids. One of the major problems with taking drugs to help you sleep is that long-term or chronic use of sleeping pills can cause addiction (in the case of drugs in the benzodiazepine class) and disturbing side effects, including abnormal sleep patterns, which actually can make insomnia worse. Also, many people complain that sleeping pills have a hangover effect the following day.

Studies in sleep laboratories show that 50 percent of all cases of insomnia are caused by psychological factors, such as depression, anxiety, and tension. Other causes include hypoglycemia (low blood sugar), too much coffee or alcohol (or both), changes in environment, pain, restless leg syndrome (an uncontrollable urge to move the legs), and fear of sleep.

SENDING YOURSELF TO SLEEP

If you are taking any prescription or over-the-counter sleep medications do not take any natural remedies without checking to make sure there are no adverse side effects.

5-HTP. 5-hydroxytryptophan induces sleep by promoting the production of serotonin in the brain.

Recommended dosage: Take 100 milligrams an hour before bedtime.

Valerian. This herb is well known as a sleep inducer due to its high content of chemicals known as valepotriates.

Recommended dosage: Take 600 milligrams an hour before bedtime.

Lavender. The essential oil of lavender is a favorite among aromatherapists for its ability to induce relaxation and sleep. Spray some on your pillow, add it to a pre-bedtime bath, or take a giant whiff directly from the bottle.

Passionflower. Many over-the-counter sleep preparations in Europe contain passionflower because it contains compounds that act like sedatives.

Recommended dosage: Take 4,000 milligrams one hour before bedtime.

Calcium and magnesium. Both of these minerals help relax the nervous system.

Recommended dosage: Take 1,500 milligrams of calcium and 750 milligrams of magnesium an hour before bedtime.

Melatonin. This hormone is secreted by the pineal gland in the brain to help regulate the body's sleep-wake cycle. Melatonin levels drop with age, so a supplement may help induce sleep.

Recommended dosage: Take 0.3 milligrams an hour before bedtime.

SENSIBLE SLEEP ADVICE

Sleeping aids—even natural ones—should be a short-term solution to sleeping problems. To avoid tossing and turning you might have to make some changes in your routine. Consider the following.

- Go to bed at the same time every night.
- Don't drink anything containing caffeine after 3 PM.
- Create a comfortable sleeping environment.
- Don't eat a late dinner and only a light snack (if you must) of bread or fruit before bedtime.
- Learn and practice relaxation techniques. Certain yoga poses are designed to promote sleep.
- Turn on soft music or focus on peaceful thoughts once you get in bed—anything that will prevent you from thinking about the stress in your life.
- Get exercise, but not at night.

WHEN TO CALL THE DOCTOR

Some people get by just fine on little sleep; others need more than the requisite eight hours. There is no doubt that you'll recognize if you have a sleeping problem because you'll feel the side effects the following day.

Consult your doctor if your insomnia lingers for more than a few weeks, or the condition begins to interfere with your feelings of physical or mental stability. Your doctor should review all prescription and over-the-counter medications you're taking to find out if they could be contributing to the problem.

If the doctor suspects a physical cause of your insomnia, you may be referred to a sleep specialist, who will monitor your sleep and brain wave patterns during the night. Your doctor will want to rule out sleep apnea, a common problem in which sleepers stop breathing for periods of 10 seconds or more several times during the night. Left untreated, apnea can potentially lead to serious health problems.

IRRITABLE BOWEL SYNDROME

Some people are irritable and grumpy by nature. The same can be said for some people's bowels. In fact, some people have bowels that are so out of sorts that doctors can't figure out what causes such havoc. But they do have a name for it: irritable bowel syndrome, or irritable bowel disease.

Irritable bowel syndrome (IBS) refers to a range of digestive complaints that can cause one or any combination of unpleasant intestinal symptoms, such as diarrhea, constipation, bloating, pain, and cramping. And it is quite common, affecting millions of Americans many of whose quality of life is either compromised or seriously disrupted by annoying or disabling symptoms.

A GUESSING GAME

IBS is what doctors call a functional disorder of the intestine, meaning there is nothing physically wrong that should make your bowels act in such a way. They also don't know what causes IBS, but stress is a major suspect. Certain foods can also aggravate a sensitive bowel. Chief among them are meat, dairy products, wheat, spicy dishes, processed foods, sugar, coffee, alcohol, and soft drinks.

Chronic IBS can lead to nutritional deficiencies, including iron, vitamin B12, folic acid, magnesium, potassium, vitamin D, and zinc. Less often low levels of vitamin K, copper, niacin, and vitamin E are seen. Correction of these deficiencies is extremely important, especially in children.

MAKING BETTER BOWELS

Multivitamin. A high-potency multivitamin–mineral supplement is recommended as part of any treatment program.

Probiotics. Acidophilus, the active culture in yogurt, aids digestion and helps keep a healthy bacterial balance in the digestive tract. Eat yogurt daily or take a supplement.
Recommended dosage: Take 1 teaspoon of acidophilus powder or liquid with water twice a day.

Peppermint. Studies show that peppermint oil helps reduce the gas and bloating associated with IBD. To be most effective, peppermint oil capsules should be enteric-coated to prevent the oil from being released in the stomach. The coating allows the oil to get to the small and large intestines.
Recommended dosage: Take 1 or 2 enteric-coated peppermint oil capsules twice a day between meals.

Psyllium. Getting enough fiber in your diet? If not, try psyllium, which is the active ingredient in natural fiber products and laxatives, such as Metamucil. Psyllium can help improve your bowel's regularity. Take according to package directions.

Ginger. Ginger comes to the rescue of a lot of digestive ailments, including IBD. Drink several cups of ginger tea throughout the day.

Chamomile. You can also try chamomile tea. Chamomile soothes and tones the digestive tract and helps ease alternating diarrhea and constipation.

PAY ATTENTION TO PREVENTION

Dietary changes can help prevent IBD outbreaks. Be mindful of what you eat. Avoid refined carbohydrates, wheat, corn, spicy foods, and popcorn. Studies have found that approximately two-thirds of people with IBS have at least one food allergy.

WHEN TO CALL THE DOCTOR

A diagnosis of IBS is made only when other suspected conditions are ruled out. There are many conditions that share symptoms similar to IBS. These include ulcerative colitis and Crohn's disease (which are grouped together as types of inflammatory bowel disease). These serious chronic inflammatory disorders always require professional care.

Other conditions that must be ruled out include celiac disease, lactose intolerance, ulcers, and infestation by a parasite, among others. In short, if you are having intestinal problems, you should see a doctor to get a proper diagnosis.

JET LAG

Waiting in an airport is a drag, but it's nothing compared to the lag you experience after a long plane ride to a different time zone.

Fly east and you'll probably have trouble getting to sleep at the new bedtime, even if you feel bone tired. Go west and you may find yourself falling asleep in a bus on your way to the next museum.

There's no question about it. Jet lag can be a real drag. In addition to fatigue, the upset to the daily rhythm of your body can interfere with your ability to concentrate, interfere with bowel regularity, and cause indigestion and headaches.

Before your next trip do some advance planning with a trip to your natural pharmacy for some herbal remedies.

JETTISON JET LAG

Siberian ginseng. You can help minimize the effects of jet travel by enhancing your body's ability to resist stress.

Recommended dosage: Two 400 milligrams of powdered root twice a day for two weeks prior to departure.

Chamomile. Sleeping pills may get you to sleep but when you are jet lagged they will leave you feeling like you have a hangover. Take some chamomile tea with you and use it at bedtime. Also take some teabags on the plane with you if you are taking an overnight flight.

Ginger. Take ginger capsules with you to offset digestive troubles.

Recommended dosage: Take two 500 milligram capsules as needed.

Eucalyptus. You don't want to be giving in to sleep in mid-day and miss out of all your vacation has to offer. If fatigue hits when you want to be awake put a few drops of eucalyptus essential oil on a tissue and take a deep breath.

KIDNEY STONES

There are a lot of things in life you can take with a grain of salt but a kidney stone—which is about the same size—is not one of them.

Anyone who's ever had a kidney stone will tell you that passing one *really, really* hurts.

A kidney stone is a hard mass composed of crystals that has separated from urine and has accumulated on the inside of the kidney. Most stones are comprised of calcium with oxalate or phosphate. Less common are stones composed of uric acid or cysteine.

Although urine contains substances that prevent the formation of crystals, these chemicals fail to do their job in some people. The painful part happens when the stone attempts to leave the kidney through the ureters, the narrow tubes that carry urine downstream.

For reasons unknown, more and more people in the United States are developing kidney stones. More than 1 million cases of kidney stones are diagnosed in the United States each year. Doctors also don't know what makes them form. Some experts believe that certain foods, such as those high in fat and low in fiber, promote the formation of kidney stones. There is evidence, however, that susceptibility to kidney stones has a lot to do with heredity.

Once a stone has formed and starts heading south, there isn't a whole lot you can do but hope that it's a nonstop trip. These are things you can do to make the trip go a lot faster and help make sure one doesn't make a return visit.

SIDE-STEPPING STONES

Saw palmetto. This herb is also called "plant cathe-ter" because it helps resolve urinary problems. Take the herb as soon as you feel the stone wanting to pass. If it doesn't pass right away, take the same amount every day until it does.

Recommended dosage: 160 milligrams a day.

Ginger. Ease the pain with a hot compress soaked in concentrated ginger tea. The compress acts as a counter-irritant to the skin.

Horsetail. This herb increases urine output. Drink it as a tea or take capsules.

Recommended dosage: 2 grams three times a day as needed.

Java. The leaves of this herb are used in Europe to treat kidney stones. Make a tea using three teaspoons of leaves per cup of water.

Lovage. This plant is a potent diuretic that is effective at helping to pass a kidney stone. Make it as a tea using two to four teaspoons of dried herb per cup of water.

Cranberry. Studies show that cranberry reduces urinary calcium levels in people with kidney stones.

Recommended dosage: 400 milligrams of standardized extract a day.

Water. Drink lots and lots of water to urge urination.

PAY ATTENTION TO PREVENTION

The most important thing you can do to prevent a kidney stone is to keep your kidneys flushing by drinking lots of water—at least 8 glasses a day. You should also follow these dietary practices.

Low-sodium. A low-salt diet will reduce the calcium in your urine, which can reduce your risk of forming new stones. Aim for 2,400 milligrams of sodium a day.

Magnesium. Studies show that this mineral helps prevent kidney stones. Eat plenty of magnesium-rich foods and take a supplement for insurance.

Recommended dosage: 800 milligrams a day.

Potassium. Studies show that people who eat lots of potassium-rich fruits and vegetables have a lower risk of getting kidney stones.

Coffee. Caffeine increases calcium in the urine, which increases the risk of forming a stone.

WHEN TO CALL THE DOCTOR

Many people can pass a kidney stone without seeing a doctor. If you do, make sure to follow up by visiting your doctor.

If you have a kidney stone and you experience other symptoms along with the pain, call your doctor. These symptoms include fever, chills, and a burning sensation during urination.

Doctors also advise urinating into a piece of gauze or cheesecloth in order to capture the stone so you can take it to the doctor. Your doctor will do an analysis to find out what type of stone it is—uric acid or calcium oxalate.

LARYNGITIS

Lost your voice? Well, the best way to get it back is to keep quiet for the next several days. But that's hardly practical, is it?

Laryngitis is an inflammation of the voice box, called the larynx, the part of the windpipe that houses the vocal cords. Overusing your voice—say, cheering all day at a football game or singing the night away—can cause hoarseness or an inability to speak at all. Sometimes smoky rooms or other irritants, a cold, or allergies can cause you to be a little hoarse.

Laryngitis generally goes away in a few days on its own, but if you don't have the time to wait, soothe your voice with these suggestions.

VOICE ACTIVATORS

Chicken broth. Actually, any soothing warm liquid will do. Fluids keep the larynx moist. Sip on warm liquids throughout the day.

Onion and honey. This is an old folk remedy for laryngitis. Put two teaspoons of onion juice in a little water and follow it with a teaspoon of honey.

Goldenseal. Herbalists use this as a gargle for laryngitis. Put a quarter teaspoon of the dried powdered herb in a cup of lukewarm water, sprinkle it with a dash of cayenne, and gargle three times a day. Be forewarned: You'll definitely notice the strong flavor.

Horehound. This herb has been used for centuries to treat laryngitis. Take it as a tea by mixing two teaspoons of dried herb with a cup of boiling water. Steep and let it cool off until it is drinkably warm. Drink three or four cups a day until your voice returns.

Plantain. This is another herb that has long been a favorite among herbalist for treating laryngitis. Mix one teaspoon in a cup of boiling water. Steep and let it cool off until it is drinkably warm.

WHEN TO CALL THE DOCTOR

If you lose your voice for no apparent reason and it is accompanied by pain and difficulty swallowing, it is a sign that something could be blocking your airways. Seek medical attention right away.

MACULAR DEGENERATION

Imagine not being able to see well enough to drive a car, watch a movie, or read a book. This is what the future looks like for people who discover that they are developing macular degeneration.

Macular degeneration is a serious eye disease and the leading cause of blindness in people over age 65. It is characterized by the loss of sharp, central vision, though peripheral vision—sight out of the corner of the eye—is not affected.

There are two forms of the disease—wet and dry. The wet form is the most severe; it comes on rapidly and causes irreversible blindness. The dry form, which progresses slowly, is the most common and affects nearly 90 percent of those with the disease—most of whom are over the age of 65. This is why doctors have another name for the condition: age-related macular degeneration (ARMD).

THE AGING EYE

ARMD occurs when drusen, cholesterol-like tiny yellow particles, begin to accumulate behind the retina and damage the photoreceptors. New research is beginning to show that drusen builds up and damages the eyes in the same way that cholesterol collects and damages the heart. In fact, there is a correlation in the incidence of macular degeneration and heart disease.

Approximately 13 million Americans have some stage of macular degeneration. At present, macular degeneration cannot be reversed, but research shows that there are ways to slow the progression and greatly reduce the risk of blindness. The same research also indicates that macular degeneration is far more preventable than once believed, even for those with a family history of the disease. In fact, you can fight macular degeneration the same way you fight heart disease.

EYE SOLUTIONS

The antioxidant formula. A few years ago the National Eye Institute completed its long-term Age-Related Eye Disease Study, which investigated the impact of nutritional therapy on the incidence and progression of macular degeneration. Researchers found that antioxidant therapy slowed progression of the disease in patients with early-stage ARMD and reduced the risk in high-risk patients. As a result, many ophthalmologists recommend taking daily supplements or a supplement formula containing these antioxidants.

- 500 milligrams of vitamin C
- 400 I.U. of vitamin E
- 15 milligrams of beta-carotene
- 80 milligrams of zinc
- 2 milligrams of cupric copper

The copper is protection against copper-deficiency anemia, which is associated with high zinc intake.

Bilberry. This herb contains antioxidants that strengthen and reinforce the collagen in the retina.

Recommended dosage: Take 100 milligrams a day.

Ginkgo. Studies show that ginkgo helps visual acuity and one study found that it might even reverse damage to the retina.

Recommended dosage: Take 80 milligrams twice a day.

WHEN TO CALL THE DOCTOR

If you detect any change in your visual acuity, contact your doctor or ophthalmologist. After age 50, it is important to have annual eye exams to detect macular degeneration—and other eye diseases—as early as possible to avoid permanent vision damage.

MEMORY LOSS

You'll pick up the whatcha-ma-call-it and deliver it to who-ze-what as soon as what's-his-name gets here to pick up you-know-who.

Do you find that your mind is having a problem getting need-at-the-moment information to the tip of your tongue fast enough for you to communicate coherently? When this happens you are experiencing benign senescent forgetfulness, or what older folks today call "a senior moment."

Like other physiological processes, your ability to retrieve information from your brain slows with age. So occasional lapses in memory are no cause for alarm. After all, you can't run as fast or work as fast as you could 20 years ago, so it should come as no surprise that you can't think as fast. However, as long as you have two good legs you can still get where you want to go, and the same can be said for your brain. Just like your body, you can keep your mind in shape by keeping it active and feeding it the nutrients it needs to keep blood flowing and your memory retrieval messaging system in top operating condition.

BRAIN FOOD

Your memory is in your brain and your brain is in your body. It lives on the same blood and nutrients as the rest of you. To be at its best, it needs the rest of you to be at its best. These nutrients can help, as long as you remember to take them!

B vitamins. A deficiency in B vitamins, especially vitamin B12, can cause memory problems. Make sure to eat plenty of B vitamin–rich foods and take a B12 supplement.

Recommended dosage: Take 800 to 1,600 micrograms of vitamin B12 a day.

Acetyl-L-carnitine. ALC is a form of carnitine that improves brain cell communication, thus improving memory.

Recommended dosage: Take 500 milligrams three times a day.

Ginkgo biloba. There are hundreds of studies to confirm the benefit of ginkgo for improving age-affected memory loss. It works by improving blood and oxygen supply to the brain.

Recommended dosage: Take up to 240 milligrams of standardized extract a day.

DHEA. Dehydroepiandrosterone is an important hormone for mental acuity. DHEA declines with age. Have your doctor check if your levels are dropping. If so consider taking DHEA supplements.

Recommended dosage: Take 15 milligrams a day.

Ginseng. This herb is associated with memory enhancement because of its ability to increase the production of DHEA.

Recommended dosage: Take 20 drops of tincture three times a day.

Ashwaganda. According to Ayurvedic medicine, ashwaganda has restorative qualities that enhance brain function, including the ability to improve memory.

Recommended dosage: Take 500 milligrams two or three times a day.

WHEN TO CALL THE DOCTOR

Forgetfulness in and of itself is not a problem, but it is if it is among a cluster of cognitive deficits that signal the onset of senile dementia. Difficulty with language, attention problems, confusion and impaired judgment are all signs of senile dementia, which is often rooted in a physical condition, such as diabetes or heart disease.

Abnormal forgetfulness (such as forgetting the name of

someone you see every day) can be a sign of early onset of Alzheimer's disease.

MENOPAUSE PROBLEMS

Menopause is a natural progression of life marking a woman's transition from the ability to have children to the horizon of new possibilities. In fact, menopause wouldn't be a problem at all if it weren't for the turmoil it can cause, both physically and emotionally.

For some women, "the change" is barely noticeable. Their periods stop and life goes on with little to complain about, except for vaginal dryness and a mild hot flash or two. At the other extreme, it can throw women into both physical and emotional turmoil, making them feel on the brink of disaster. All this trouble is caused by out-of-sync hormones, which are going every which way in an effort to make a final exit. The discomforts can be especially severe if menstruation stops abruptly, either naturally or following the surgical removal of the ovaries.

WHEN CHANGE IS NOT SO GOOD

The most complex physical symptom of menopause is a hot flash, which can come on almost without notice, creating an internal fire that results in flushing and profuse sweating. Hot flashes are often the most troublesome at night.

Hot flashes happen when estrogen levels drop, which causes a sudden adjustment in the body's thermostat and an abrupt "flash" of heat. (The pituitary gland in the brain controls both estrogen levels and body temperature, hence the link between hormones and heat.)

Typically, the heat of a hot flash begins in the chest and

spreads to the neck, face, and arms. It can be followed by chills.

Three out of four menopausal women experience hot flashes, which can occur as often as once an hour and last for three or four minutes at a stretch. For most women, hot flashes are mild and end within two years, but 25 percent of women who experience hot flashes suffer from them for more than five years, and about 10 percent "flash" for the rest of their lives.

Other symptoms of menopause include heart palpitations, insomnia, headaches, bladder control problems, fatigue, and changes in the skin. Some women suffer mentally from depression, anxiety, and mood swings.

At one time doctors believed that the cure-all for all menopause-related problems was to prolong the body's hormone dependency with synthetic hormone replacement therapy (HRT). This brewed lots of controversy, including an increased risk of cancer so alarming that a major clinical trial to measure the effects of HRT on breast cancer was terminated.

Long before HRT, however, women managed menopause with natural therapies and many women are doing it again.

ADJUSTING THE TIME CLOCK

Black cohosh. Studies have found that the estrogenlike qualities of this herb can relieve a variety of menopausal symptoms, most notably hot flashes.

Recommended dosage: Take 80 milligrams once or twice a day, depending on your symptoms.

Flaxseed. A preliminary study at the Mayo Clinic found that women who took flaxseed every day for six weeks experienced a 50 percent reduction in hot flashes. Flaxseed has estrogenlike qualities. Try adding flaxseed to your diet.

Soy foods. Soy contains phytoestrogens, which are similar to the estrogen women manufacture in the body. Studies show that women who eat soy foods on a regular basis have fewer hot flashes. They also have more cells in the vaginal lining, which helps reduce irritation and dryness. In addition to eating soy, you can take soy protein powder. Follow the package directions.

Chasteberry. This herb has complex biochemistry actions that balance the hormonal system.

Recommended dosage: Take 500 to 1,000 milligrams a day.

Red clover. If eating soy foods is not your preference, try red clover, which also contains phytoestrogens.

Recommended dosage: Take 370 milligrams twice a day.

Wild yam. The root of this plant contains diosgenin, which is similar to estrogen and progesterone. In fact, until 1970, this plant was used in the manufacture of birth control pills. While the body does not covert wild yam into estrogen, the plant's active ingredients can help relieve menopausal symptoms. Take according to package directions.

Vitamin E. Studies show that taking vitamin E can help control hot flashes in some women.

Recommended dosage: Take 400 I.U. a day.

Estriol cream. This is a natural lubricant that can help relieve vaginal dryness. Use it nightly for two weeks, then as needed.

WHEN TO CALL THE DOCTOR

One out of every two women experiences some symptoms associated with menopause, and about one in four find them anywhere from uncomfortable to distressing. If the symptoms of menopause interfere with your quality of life, consult your doctor.

MOTION SICKNESS

The sky is blue, the sea is green, and you're a pasty gray. The listing and lobbing and crashing and splashing are churning your stomach and sinking your day. Motion sickness has got you again—and it's not going to be a pretty.

Motion sickness is an odd condition in which you can be miserably sick for hours and feel better the moment you step foot on land.

Though it feels like all the turmoil is centered in your digestive system, motion sickness has nothing to do with the stomach. It is really a problem with the inner ear, which regulates balance. Normally when the eyes sense motion they send a signal to the inner ear to keep the body in balance. For some reason, even mild rocking can send a miscue to the inner ear, which puts your equilibrium off keel and starts your stomach rolling.

Any kind of motion—boat, airplane, car, Ferris wheel—can cause this worse-than-death, sick-all-over feeling. Unfortunately, once you've got it there isn't a whole lot you can do except get yourself on firm ground, if you can, or ride it out.

If you've had motion sickness once, you don't have to get it again. Here's what you can do to help weather the next storm.

MOTION DETECTORS

Ginger. Take it in whatever form you desire—candy, capsule, fresh, or as a soda. Ginger is a powerful antidote to motion sickness. One study found that ginger capsules are as effective as some motion sickness medications.

Recommended dosage: Take 250 milligrams to prevent motion sickness.

The mints. Peppermint and spearmint are prime scents

for the overwhelming nausea of motion sickness. Take a strong whiff from a vial of essential oil.

Lemon. At the first hint of nausea, suck on a lemon. It can help calm your stomach by dissolving excess saliva, which contributes to your sickly feeling.

Soda crackers. Food may be the last thing you want, but bland soda crackers can do the same thing a lemon does but even better.

Coke syrup. This is an old-time cure doctors often recommended during the days when soda fountains were common. The next best thing to the syrup is a flat Coke.

Diet. Avoid fatty and fried foods and alcohol. If you should get motion sickness, these foods will make it all the worse.

OSTEOARTHRITIS

Arthritis may be the oldest ailment known to mankind. Archeologists have detected it in mummies, prehistoric human remains, and even dinosaur bones.

You could say that arthritis is a fact of life. If you live long enough, you're going to get it. Only thing is, some people are going to get it sooner and more severely than others. To a great degree, it all depends on you.

Like anything else—a car, a toy, or a piece of furniture—time and use take a toll on the body. Outwardly it shows up as gray hair, wrinkles, and a few sags here and there. Inwardly, you start to notice it in your joints. Maybe you can't sit cross-legged or bend over without feeling discomfort on the way back up. Perhaps you lack the grip you once had to open a jar. It may be too painful to swing a racket, work with your hands, or even move your hips. It doesn't take a doctor to tell you that these are all signs of osteoarthritis.

Arthritis comes in many forms, but osteoarthritis is the most common—and the most inevitable. Some 40 million Americans are living with age-related joint pain. By age 60, most people have some hints of arthritis but it can start in the 50s and even 40s. Osteoarthritis can also develop prematurely as a result of an injury, trauma, physical abnormality in the joint, or a previous joint disease.

GETTING OUT OF JOINT

The human joint is like a well-oiled hinge. A layer of cartilage covers the ends of the bones, and a membrane inside the joint secretes a lubricating gel known as synovial fluid. An outer shell or joint capsule surrounds the various components of the joint and keeps them intact. This system works remarkably well. In a healthy joint, the bones glide back and forth and allow movement without grinding or rubbing bone against bone.

As you age, cartilage in the joints starts to wear, especially in the fingers, hips, knees, and spine. This causes inflammation, pain, and restriction in range of motion. In many cases, the synovial fluid starts to thin and bone joints can rub together, causing stiffness or intense pain. Cartilage at the ends of the bones can also wear away, causing additional pain.

There is some belief that this breakdown in cartilage is, at least in part, caused by the lack of sufficient glucosamine, a substance involved in the structural health of cartilage. Glucosamine in the body diminishes with age.

There are plenty of anti-inflammatory and prescription medications that can ease the pain or arthritis. Unfortunately, they all have side effects. One popular arthritis medication even had to be taken off the market.

Short of surgically getting an artificial joint, you can't do much about the damage that has already taken place. But there is a lot you can do to slow down and even stop the progression of arthritis.

JOINT PROGRESS

Glucosamine and chondroitin. These two substances are major players in building and maintaining the cartilage that surrounds the joints. Chondroitin is specifically involved in the fluid environment that protects the joints. Both substances diminish with age. Many studies have confirmed the effectiveness of this two supplements in diminishing pain and increasing the quality of life for people with arthritis. The substances are manufactured together specifically for joint health. Be patient. It can take several months until you notice a change.

Recommended dosage: Take 1,500 milligrams of glucosamine and 1,200 milligrams of chondroitin sulfate a day.

Fish oil. Fish oil is a direct source of omega-3 fatty acids, which reduces joint pain and promotes joint lubrication.

Recommended dosage: Take a supplement containing 1.8 milligrams of DHA and 1.2 milligrams of EPA a day.

Capsaicin. This substance that puts the hotness in cayenne pepper triggers the release of the body's natural pain-relieving chemicals. Use it as a topical ointment to relieve pain.

Bromelain. The chemical component of pineapple helps the body get rid of immune antigen compounds that are associated with arthritis.

Recommended dosage: Take 500 milligrams three times a day.

Boron. German doctors have been using boron supplements to treat osteoarthritis since the mid-1970s. One study found a 70 percent improvement in people taking 6 milligrams of boron a day. Look for a multivitamin supplement containing boron or consider taking a boron supplement.

Recommended dosage: Take 6 to 9 milligrams a day.

Ginger. Studies have found ginger useful in providing pain relief, decreasing swelling and stiffness in the joints, and increasing joint mobility in people with osteoarthritis.

Recommended dosage: Take 500 milligrams a day.

PAY ATTENTION TO PREVENTION

The "use it or lose it" prescription applies here. Exercise helps keep bones and joints healthy. Weight-bearing exercise, such as using light weights, builds strong muscles that, in turn, support the joints and absorb shock.

Being overweight is hard on the joints. The more excess weight you carry, the greater the likelihood that you will develop osteoarthritis. Think about it: If you injured your knee, would you want to lug around a 25-pound bag of sand all day? To your knees, there's no difference between 25 pounds of fat and 25 pounds of sand.

OSTEOPOROSIS

If it hadn't been for her bleeped Emmy-winning acceptance speech, Sally Field might be better known for her role as the osteoporosis poster child.

Her public image as an older woman with osteoporosis is more than a reminder to take a pill; it's also a subliminal message that taking care of your bones should start much sooner than the sixth decade of life. It's a lifetime job.

Osteoporosis means porous, or brittle, bones. And it has quality-of-life consequences. It makes you fragile. It puts you at high risk for bone fractures, especially of the hip. We often hear of an older woman who "fell and broke a hip." What's really happening is, "she broke a hip and fell." In advanced cases, a good cough can break a rib, or a gentle bump can fracture a hip. In fact, nearly half a million older people every year end up with a broken hip as a result of osteoporosis.

It is estimated that one out of every three women over age 60 has osteoporosis. Men get it, too, but it is less common and less severe, in part because men start out with denser bones than women do.

BONE–CALCIUM CONNECTION

Calcium is the most abundant mineral in the body and about 99 percent of it resides in our bones. The other 1 percent roams around the bloodstream to help maintain vital processes, like regulating the heartbeat and making muscles contract. The blood needs calcium, so when the supply dwindles, it steals it from the bones. This begins to become a problem after the bones reach peak mass. Typically, this happens around age 30 for the spine and around age 35 for the long bones. After that, bone mass starts to decline by about 1 percent a year.

In women, however, menopause causes bone loss to accelerate. This is due to the decline in the female hormone estrogen, which helps the body absorb calcium. For every 10 percent loss in bone mass, the risk of bone fracture doubles. By the age of 80, most women have lost from a quarter to half of their bone mass.

As the disease progresses, the spinal column starts to compress, causing the characteristic curve known as a dowager's hump. These spinal changes actually result from fractures caused by the pressure of the body's weight on weak and brittle bones.

In addition to dietary calcium deficiency, osteoporosis can also be caused by the inability to absorb enough calcium through the intestine or a calcium-phosphorus imbalance.

Women at highest risk are those with a thin frame, a sedentary lifestyle, family history of the disease, and those who surgically reach menopause before the age of 40. Smoking, alcohol, caffeine also increase risk because they inhibit the body's ability to absorb calcium. Certain drugs, such as cortisone, anticoagulants, anticonvulsants, and thyroid medications can also contribute to calcium loss.

These natural treatment options can help prevent osteoporosis and slow its progression.

BONE BUILDERS

Calcium. There isn't a woman over age 40 who hasn't been told to make sure to get enough calcium. In perimenopausal women, studies show that calcium supplementation can help delay osteoporosis later in life. In postmenopausal women, long-term studies show that calcium supplementation can slow the rate of calcium loss by at least 30 to 50 percent and significantly protect against hip fractures.

Recommended dosage: Take 600 milligrams twice a day.

Vitamin D. Calcium depends on the sunshine vitamin to help absorption. If you wear sunscreen or do not get sufficient exposure to the sun for other reasons, you might benefit from vitamin D supplementation. A good multivitamin–mineral supplement should contain 400 I.U. daily, which is all you need.

Magnesium. The mineral is also important to calcium absorption.

Recommended dosage: Take 250 milligrams twice a day with calcium.

Boron. This mineral activates vitamin D and improves estrogen levels. It also helps the body absorb calcium, magnesium and phosphorus. A study of postmenopausal women conducted by the U.S. Department of Agriculture found that supplementing their diet with 3 milligrams of boron for eight days prevented the loss of essential bone nutrients. They lost 40 percent less calcium, one-third less magnesium, and slightly less phosphorus through their urine than they had before beginning boron supplementation.

Recommended dosage: Take 3 to 5 milligrams daily as sodium tetrahydroborate or sodium tetraborate decahydrate.

Horsetail. This herb is the richest plant source of silicon, which gives bones strength and flexibility. Research indicates that aging plus declining estrogen levels decrease the body's natural stores of silicon.

Recommended dosage: 350 milligrams a day.

PAY ATTENTION TO PREVENTION

The best way to prevent osteoporosis is follow a healthy lifestyle that builds strong bones early in life and maintains them for the rest of your life. This includes the following

- Getting enough calcium. Studies show that the average American woman does not get enough calcium through food to maintain healthy bones. Women should get between 1,200–1,500 milligrams a day.
- Getting enough exercise. Weight-bearing exercise is particularly good for maintaining strong bones.
- Don't smoke.
- Keep consumption of alcohol, caffeine, and carbonated beverages to a minimum.
- Get 15 minutes of exposure to the sun every day. In summer, go out early in the morning when the sun is not as strong.

OVERWEIGHT

Obesity is a big fat thief. It drains your emotional life, limits your active life, diminishes your social life, and takes from your quality of life. Worst of all, it robs you of life itself.

Obesity can cut 20 years from your life span. It is second only to smoking as the leading cause of death and is the major risk factor in a number of life-threatening diseases, including cancer, diabetes, stroke, and heart disease.

Obesity is defined as being 20 percent or more over your ideal weight, but any amount of excess weight jeopardizes your health. A recent study found that being even moderately overweight increases the risk of heart disease *independent* of all other risk factors. Excess weight also increases blood pressure, contributes to varicose veins, and makes you more prone to gallbladder disease, hemorrhoids, kidney disease, and liver problems. In women, it contributes to infertility and makes the symptoms of premenstrual syndrome worse.

IT'S EPIDEMIC

There is a lot of irony in the fact that a nation that reveres thinness is also gaining weight at record speed. A record two-thirds of all Americans adults and 15 percent of children are overweight. If the trend continues, the Centers for Disease Control and Prevention predicts that life expectancy for future generations will decline for the first time in history.

The root cause of this phenomenon is the subject of much debate and study among bariatricians, epidemiologists, psychologists, and sociologists. And there is plenty to ponder: On any given day nearly 50 percent of Americans (mostly women) are trying some kind of diet; meanwhile, we're eating more (average daily caloric intake is at an all-time high) and exercising less.

THE DIET DILEMMA

Food supplies the body with energy, which is defined in units called calories. One pound of body weight is equal to

2,800 calories. When you eat 2,800 calories more than you burn, you gain. Eat 2,800 less, you lose. So the theory goes.

Yet we all know thin people who eat like prizefighters and don't gain a pound. What's going on? Why do some people burn fat fast and other store fat fast? There are lots of theories, but as yet no breakthrough discoveries that work for *all* people. However, there is a lot of evidence that the bodies of thin people and fat people don't work alike. Do heavy people possess or lack a natural substance that is making them fat? Is some biochemical process out of sync that is messing up their metabolisms?

There are hundreds of diet books and dozens of pills on the market that claim to be the answer to weight loss. Many have some degree of success. Here is what is most promising from the standpoint of natural health.

WINNERS AT LOSING

CLA. Several studies that taking supplemental conjugated linoleic acid, a slightly altered fatty acid derived from meat and dairy, can lead to weight loss success. Researchers believe that CLA increases metabolism and decreases fat absorption by blocking fat-storing enzymes.

Recommended dosage: Take 3 grams a day.

5-HTP. The amino acid 5-hydroxytryptophan acts as a weight loss suppressant by increasing levels of serotonin in the brain. Serotonin is the so-called "hunger switch" that turns on satiety. Studies found that overweight women who took 5-HTP ate fewer calories and lost weight.

Recommended dosage: Take 100 to 300 milligrams three times a day.

Green tea. Studies show that the polyphenols in green tea and green tea extract promote weight loss by increasing the rate at which the body burns fat. In one three-month study, green tea reduced weight an average of 4.5 percent and waist circumference by 4.4 percent.

Guarana. This South American caffeine-containing herb is best known for enhancing endurance but it is also associated with weight loss. One study found that people who took guarana extract for 45 days lost an average of 11 pounds. Guarana can have adverse side effects, so take it only under the guidance of a doctor or qualified weight loss specialist.

Chromium. Chromium is involved in glucose tolerance and can help reduce sweet cravings. In one study, volunteers were given either chromium supplements or a placebo for 72 days; they were not given any diet or exercise regimen. Those taking chromium lost an average of 4.2 pounds of fat and gained 1.4 pounds of lean muscle mass. There was little change in those taking the placebo. Other studies have found that the chromium's weight loss benefit is greatest in people with a chromium deficiency and the elderly.

Recommended dosage: Take 200 to 400 micrograms of chromium picolinate daily.

Psyllium. This natural fiber supplement can help produce weight loss by increasing feelings of satiety. Stir half to 1 teaspoon psyllium powder or husks in 8 ounces of water and drink 2 cups a day. Do not take any other supplement or medications at the same time.

Spirulina. One study found that people who took 8 grams of supplemental blue-green algae known as spirulina lost weight. Look for a spirulina supplement geared to weight loss and take according to package directions.

Stevia. If you have a sweet tooth you can help reduce calories by using stevia in place of sugar. Stevia is a natural sweetener that is sold as a dietary supplement in natural food stores.

PAY ATTENTION TO PREVENTION

This begins with paying attention to the scale. Weigh yourself regularly. When the bathroom scale shows you weigh five pounds more than your goal weight, it's time to reduce your food intake and increase your activity level. These sensible practices also will help you maintain a healthy weight.

Avoid trans fats. These fats, which have the peculiar ability to stay solid at room temperature, are man-made; therefore, the body does not recognize them. As a result, some scientists believe, the body stores them as fat rather than turning them into a ready form of energy. This is why many speculate that fast and processed foods are core to the current obesity problem in the United States.

Eat nine servings of fruits and vegetables a day. They are low in fat and calories and also good at preventing a host of diseases. Eating lots of fruits and vegetables will help fill you up so you will naturally cut down on your intake of high-fat foods.

Drink lots of water. Water helps keep the body hydrated, it helps with metabolism—and it's filling. Try drinking a glass of water before you sit down to a meal if you feel you might be tempted to overindulge. Drink at least 8 glasses of water a day.

Eat slowly. It can take 20 minutes for your brain to recognize that your stomach feels full.

Keep a food diary. Studies show that the most successful weight loss strategy used by people who have successfully lost weight and kept it off is keeping a daily diary of everything you eat.

WHEN TO CALL THE DOCTOR

Anyone who has ever tried to diet knows how difficult it is to lose weight. If you have a weight problem, seek professional advice from a nutritionist or qualified weight loss center.

You should also discuss the problem with your primary care physician. It is possible there is a physical factor involved in your weight problem that has nothing to do with your diet, such as low serotonin levels in the brain, impaired metabolism, glandular malfunctions, a food allergy, or sensitivity to insulin.

PARKINSON'S DISEASE

It's not easy living in a body with Parkinson's disease. Muscles in one part of the body may freeze up while others contract involuntarily. Someone with Parkinson's disease may stoop, shuffle, and appear stone-faced, while at the same time shake from an incessant tremor in the hand.

Parkinson's is a degenerative disorder of the nervous system that affects voluntary movement. Parkinson's is caused by a malfunction in small sections of the brain called basal cell ganglia that coordinate the body's internal communication system. Every movement we make, be it kicking a ball or writing a letter, requires thousands of coordinated signals between the brain, muscles, tendons, and nerve cells. This system is dependent on two neurotransmitters, acetylcholine and dopamine, that work in tandem to regulate muscle movement. Acetylcholine helps muscle contract and dopamine helps keep movement fluid.

In a healthy body, this system works so well we can move about without giving it any thought. But when the network breaks down, it results in the devastating effects of Parkinson's disease. This happens when neurons that secrete dopamine gradually start to die. As dopamine supply in the brain dwindles, the symptom of Parkinson's become more pronounced. Why this happens is still a medical mystery.

SHAKING PALSY

Once known simply as shaking palsy, British physician James Parkinson identified the disease in 1817. While much has been learned about the disease over these many years, both a cause and a cure still elude medical science. However, there is some evidence that environmental toxins, including pesticides, insecticides, carbon monoxide, and recreational drugs, can influence the onset.

More than 1 million Americans are afflicted with Parkinson's. It progresses slowly—generally over a period of 10 or 15 years—and usually strikes in the 60s or 70s. However, cases of younger people getting Parkinson's is becoming more common, as is the well-known case of actor Michael J. Fox, who has been battling the disease most of his adult life.

Parkinson's is a serious disease that requires medical supervision. The most common therapy is the drug levodopa (L-dopa), which is taken up and converted to dopamine. It's been proven to alleviate the symptoms and slow the progression of the disease. There are also some natural therapies that can help assist the medication. If you're considering taking any of them, make sure to discuss it with your doctor and take them only under medical supervision.

MUSCLE MOVERS

NADH. Nicotinamide adenine dinucleotide is the focus of much of the research on a natural approach to treating Parkinson's. The brain uses NADH to manufacture neurotransmitters and create chemical activity in the brain. It is also an active form of niacin, a B vitamin important to brain health. NADH levels decrease with age. Preliminary research is showing modest results in Parkinson's patients.

Recommended dosage: Take 5 milligrams twice a day.

Calcium and magnesium. These minerals work in tandem to support a healthy nervous system.

Recommended dosage: Take 1,000 milligrams of calcium and 500 milligrams of magnesium.

Vitamin C. Vitamin C is an important detoxifier that fights free radical damage from environmental pollutants. One study showed that 60 percent of the elderly people with vitamin C deficiency had Parkinson's disease.

Recommended dosage: Take 3,000 milligrams divided throughout the day.

Vitamin E. This antioxidant is beneficial for the same reasons as vitamin C.

Recommended dosage: Take 400 I.U. daily.

Ginkgo biloba. Ginkgo is a brain aid because it helps improve blood flow. It also aids in the delivering system that transmits dopamine.

Recommended dosage: Take 300 to 500 milligrams of standardized ginkgo extract containing 25 percent flavonoids.

WHEN TO CALL THE DOCTOR

Unfortunately, the early warning signs of Parkinson's include vague symptoms that are often written off as typical signs of aging, including fatigue, stiffness, and slight hand tremor.

Classic Parkinson's symptoms—such as a constant "pill-rolling" motion of the fingers, a tendency to hold an arm with the elbow bent, a change in handwriting, and a "mask-like" expression—tend to show up next. Finally, more severe signs appear, such as a slow, shuffling walk, severe tremor, stooped posture, muscle rigidity, and dementia.

You should see your doctor at the first sign of any of these symptoms. In some cases people develop symptoms of Parkinson's disease that turn out to be side effects of medication. This is called Parkinson's syndrome rather than Parkinson's disease, and the symptoms disappear when the drugs are discontinued.

PNEUMONIA

Pneumonia can be a threat to your life because it gets you when you're already down. It is a serious infection and one of the leading causes of death in the United States.

Pneumonia burrows deep in the lungs of people with immune systems already weakened by other health-related problems, but most cases result from just two sources—the flu or a hospital-acquired infection. But anyone with an immune system compromised by chronic disease can get pneumonia. Elderly people who are hospitalized or in a nursing home are at the highest risk for dying from pneumonia.

Any kind of germ—bacteria, fungus, protozoa, or virus—can cause pneumonia and it is usually the kind that normally wouldn't bother you if your immune system weren't so depleted.

Pneumonia is actually an infection of the alveoli, the tiny air sacs that transfer oxygen from the lungs to the blood. When mild, pneumonia can be mistaken for a cold. In more serious cases, it can put you to bed for days with a rib-rattling cough, fever, and the chills.

Pneumonia is a serious illness that should be treated by a

physician, though you can also use natural remedies to help manage your symptoms.

IMMUNE BOOSTERS

Beta-carotene. Research shows that people who have low blood levels of beta-carotene and vitamin A (beta-carotene is a form of vitamin A) have an increased risk of respiratory infections and pneumonia.

Recommended dosage: Take 10,000 I.U. a day.

Vitamin C. This inflammation fighter helps protect the airways.

Recommended dosage: Take 1,000 milligrams three times a day.

Astragalus. This root is used by Chinese doctors to treat infections.

Recommended dosage: 100–150 milligrams solid extract three times a day.

Echinacea. This is one of the best immune-boosting herbs. Herbalists recommend it for all kinds of infections.

Recommended dosage: Take 500 milligrams as a capsule four times a day.

Garlic. You can enhance the effects of echinacea with garlic. Get the equivalent of 6–10 cloves a day through diet or capsules.

Sundew. German herbalists use sundew to treat bacterial pneumonia.

Recommended dosage: Take 2 teaspoons of tincture a day.

PAY ATTENTION TO PREVENTION

Anyone can get a cold or the flu but it never has to lead to pneumonia. Also, bronchitis, which affects the gateway to the lungs, is just a short trip from pneumonia.

If you have a cold, flu or bronchitis, follow the advice for these conditions found in this book. You can find how to care for a cold and the flu on page 91 and bronchitis on page 64.

WHEN TO CALL THE DOCTOR

Symptoms of pneumonia include fever, chills, cough, muscle aches, swollen lymph glands, fatigue, sore throat, chest pains, and difficulty breathing. If you have a respiratory infection in which the symptoms get worse in spite of treatment, call the doctor.

PREMENSTRUAL SYNDROME

Premenstrual syndrome is like a war of sex hormones waged once a month in a women's reproductive system.

On one side is estrogen and on the other, progesterone. They get along pretty peaceably most of the time, except the time of month when they are called into action to do the fertility dance. They move up, down, and even a little out of harmony, which is okay—but only to a point. Problem is, progesterone, which exists primarily to support pregnancy, wants to be top dog in this act but estrogen sometimes takes over and even dominates. It can also happen the other way around. Either way, they take it out on *you*—and you feel the brunt of it through any of a large array of symptoms.

HORMONES OUT OF SYNC

Premenstrual syndrome, or PMS as it is familiarly known, is not a condition but a cluster of uncomfortable symptoms that many women experience one to two weeks before the onset of menstruation. It has only been recognized as a syndrome for about 50 years; before that the out-of-sorts symptoms were just considered normal female biological behavior. But not all women experience premenstrual woes and those who do experience different symptoms at different degrees of severity.

Something like 150 different PMS symptoms have been identified. Some of the more common ones include fatigue, irritability, depression, headache, nervousness, anxiety, mood swings, abdominal bloating, diarrhea, constipation, cravings for sugar, tender and enlarged beasts, uterine cramping, altered sex drive, backache, acne, and swelling of the ankles and fingers.

An estimated 40 percent of women experience PMS to some degree and many have found success in alleviating symptoms from one or more of these natural remedies. Choose the options that match your symptoms.

PMS CHASERS

Calcium. Studies show calcium supplements help improve a variety of symptoms characteristic of PMS. In one study, 500 women with PMS took 1,200 milligrams of calcium (as calcium carbonate) for three months. They reported a reduction in moodiness, water retention, food cravings, and cramps.

Recommended dosage: Take 1,500 milligrams daily in divided dosages.

Magnesium. This mineral, which is involved in regulating estrogen, has been found to be helpful in relieving menstrual cramps.

Recommended dosage: Take 250 milligrams a day as needed.

Vitamin B6. Pyridoxine helps relieves depression associated with PMS. It also helps magnesium absorption.

Recommended dosage: Take 50 milligrams one or two times a day.

Vitamin E. This vitamin helps relieve breast tenderness, headache, fatigue, and nervous tension associated with PMS. In a study of 75 women treated for 2 months with vitamin E, 75 percent reported improvement in their PMS symptoms.

Recommended dosage: Take 400 I.U. a day.

Chasteberry. This herb has been used since ancient times for menstrual disorders because of its ability to help balance hormones. Women who are prone to depression should not take it.

Recommended dosage: Take 180 to 240 milligrams of standardized extract a day.

Dandelion. This herb acts as a mild diuretic and can help water retention associated with PMS.

Recommended dosage: Take 300 milligrams three times a day before the start of your cycle.

Evening primrose oil. The leaves and flowers of the evening primrose plant contain a valuable oil that helps relieve a variety of PMS symptoms including cramps, depression, and breast tenderness.

Recommended dosage: Take 500 milligrams twice daily.

Dong quai. Known as female ginseng, dong quai is a species of the angelica plant that helps relieve painful cramps.

Recommended dosage: Take 300 to 500 milligrams twice a day beginning a week prior to the onset of menstruation.

DIET AIDS

Some women report that PMS symptoms get worse when they eat poorly and improve when they eat healthfully. Here are some dietary recommendations to ease PMS.

- Decrease your intake of high-fat foods and salty foods, especially around the time you are expecting your period.

- Avoid overeating. Rather, eat smaller meals more often throughout the day.
- Eat high fiber foods that are complex carbohydrates, such as vegetables and beans.
- Avoid spicy foods, high-acid foods, and caffeine, which can aggravate symptoms.

WHEN TO CALL THE DOCTOR

If your PMS symptoms interfere with your relationships and quality of life, talk to your doctor about it. You may need some clinical tests to rule out other hormone imbalances that may be contributing to your condition.

PROSTATE PROBLEMS

Sometimes bigger isn't always better. The prostate is a case in point.

The prostate is a walnut-sized gland and the semen-manufacturing site of the male reproductive system. It fits snugly just below the bladder and in front of the rectum and encircles the upper part of the urethra, the tube that transports urine from the bladder.

Sooner or later, most men will know what it's like to have an enlarged prostate. It happens to around 10 to 15 percent of men by age 45. By age 80, 90 percent of men will have experienced the discomfort of an enlarged prostate. There is even a name for it: benign prostatic hyperplasia, or BPH.

ALL TUCKED IN AND NO WAY TO GO

The problem with BPH is that it makes urination a problem, especially at night. The urge is there but the spill isn't. When the prostate is enlarged, it squeezes the prostatic urethra, which makes urination difficult. For some men it can go on all night, causing disruptive sleep and all the problems associated with it. Many men with enlarged prostates experience painful urination, or a feeling that the bladder is never empty. Often, an enlarged prostate can cause a weak urinary stream. The problem eventually causes enough distress to send a man to the doctor seeking a solution. This is smart because difficult urination can lead to other problems, including kidney infection or an infection of the prostate gland itself.

FROM BAD TO WORSE

If urine is not completely emptied, it leaves both the prostate and kidneys open to infection from fungus, viruses, microbes, or bacteria. The prostate becomes tender and inflamed and leads to the full range of infectious symptoms: fever, back pain, chills, painful urination, and possibly even blood in the urine. The telltale sign that it could be prostatitis: tenderness in the area between the genitals and the anus.

Depending on the cause, prostatitis can be hard to treat, even with antibiotics. This can lead to a chronic condition. Though rare, it can result in removal of the prostate.

Another condition that threatens the life of the prostate is cancer. Prostate cancer is the most common cancer in men. In fact here's the bad news: If you live long enough, it is bound to get you. By age 50 the chance of getting prostate cancer is 30 percent and it rises to 80 percent by age 90. Prostate cancer is slow growing. This doesn't mean, however, that it isn't deadly.

Now for the good news: Prostate cancer can be detected early and therefore treated effectively through a simple test called prostate specific antigen (PSA). A PSA test should be part of a man's annual physical examination starting at age 40.

There are many successful treatment options available today that do not require the radical removal of the prostate. Some don't involve surgery at all. If you are diagnosed with prostate cancer, especially in the early stages, it is always a good idea to get a second opinion from a doctor whose treatment of choice is nonsurgical.

HOW PROBLEMS BEGIN

As men age, hormone balance changes, just as it does in women. Testosterone levels decline and a form of estrogen called estradiol increases. One theory behind age-onset prostate trouble involves the increased conversion of testosterone into one of its metabolites, dihydrotestosterone (DHT). Some research shows that the balance among estrogen, testosterone, and DHT is the source of prostate growth. Dietary and environmental toxins are also linked to prostate disease. It is interesting to note that pesticides, herbicides, and other environmental pollutants mimic estrogen in the body.

This is all the more reason to practice preventive care. Many of the steps you can take to prevent prostate health can also heal a troubled prostate.

FOODS FOR PROSTATE HEALTH

Lycopene. You'll never feel guilty for eating pizza again! There are more than 70 studies that show a link between intake of lycopene and a reduced risk of prostate cancer. Lycopene is a superrich carotenoid abundant in tomatoes. To get the maximum benefit from tomatoes, forego the raw tomato in favor of tomato products because cooking enhances lycopene. In fact, the foods most abundant in lycopene are tomato sauce, tomato juice, and pizza sauce. There is still not enough evidence that lycopene supplements are as effective as tomato-based foods. However, man cannot live on pizza and spaghetti. Consider a supplement.

Recommended dosage: 15 milligrams a day.

Strawberries. One study found that men who ate a half-cup of strawberries a day had a 20 percent reduced risk of prostate cancer. Researchers believe the source of protection comes from a substance called lupeol, which is involved in the synthesis of testosterone.

Pomegranate. One study of 50 men with recurring prostate cancer found that drinking 8 ounces of pomegranate juice a day significantly slowed the progression of the new growth. Researchers conjecture that drinking pomegranate juice could possibly be a viable treatment in older men with the disease.

Pumpkin seeds. Chewing on pumpkin seeds is the more traditional dietary therapy for a healthy prostate. Pumpkin seeds are an excellent source of zinc.

THE SUPPLEMENTAL APPROACH

Saw palmetto. This herb works by inhibiting the process that turns testosterone into dihydrotestosterone, improving urinary flow.

Recommended dosage: 160 milligrams of extract standardized to 85 to 95 percent fatty acids twice a day.

Zinc. Zinc helps reduce an enlarged prostate. It is also used to assist therapy for prostatitis.

Recommended dosage: 100 milligrams a day for an inflamed or enlarged prostate or 50 milligrams a day for general prostate health.

Stinging Nettle. Studies show that taking this herb can decrease the nighttime urge to urinate.

Recommended dosage: 300 to 600 milligrams of the root extract daily.

Beta-sistosterol. One study involving 200 men found that supplemental beta-sistosterol improved problems associated with BPH, most notably nighttime urination. Beta-sistosterol is a plant sterol, similar in structure to cholesterol.

Recommended dosage: 60 milligrams a day.

WHEN TO CALL THE DOCTOR

If you experience the symptoms of prostatitis—pain during urination, discharge from the penis, and fever—contact your doctor. You may need antibiotics or other medicines to clear the condition. In addition, if you experience urinary difficulty that affects your quality of life, discuss the matter with your doctor; in some cases, surgery is required to treat BPH.

You should also have a yearly PSA test as a guard against prostate cancer.

PSORIASIS

Psoriasis is like a traffic jam of the skin. When everything is running normally—that is, new skin cells following old skin cells—the skin's surface is smooth and clear. When new cells are generated too quickly, they get in the way of other skin cells that are not quite ready to move on. This is what causes the jam. When new cells can't get to the surface of the skin, they start to pile up like a chain collision on a freeway.

Psoriasis is an autoimmune disease in which skin cells replicate at an accelerated speed, causing thick, red, scaly patches on the skin. It can also be extremely itchy. The condition can show up anywhere on the skin but the most common sites are the scalp, elbows, knees, back, and buttocks.

While we can identify with a traffic jam, scientists have yet to identify the cause of psoriasis. There are several theories, however, that point to diet. Some researchers say that a high-fat diet is involved because psoriasis is rare in areas of the world where a low-fat diet is the norm. Others say that the type of fat eaten is more important than the amount: It appears that people who do not get enough dietary essential fatty acids are more prone to the skin condition. Another theory holds that psoriasis is the result of an accumulation of toxins in the intestinal tract. There is a lot of evidence of a genetic link, as well.

Some people with psoriasis have a hard time digesting protein and fatty foods, such as red meat and milk. These two foods also contain arachidonic acid, which can cause a flare-up.

There is no cure for psoriasis, so the best treatment is trying to avoid flare-ups. Triggers associated with psoriasis include stress, illness or any trauma to the skin, sunburn, alcohol, and certain medications such as nonsteroidal anti inflammatory drugs.

THE ROAD TO SMOOTHER SKIN

Milk thistle. Herbalists recommend milk thistle as a treatment because it has a reputation for protecting and repairing liver cells. The liver plays a crucial role in eliminating toxins from the body.

Recommended dosage: 100 milligrams of standardized extract three times day.

Vitamin A. This vitamin plans a crucial role in keeping skin healthy. Vitamin A is fat soluble and can be toxic at high levels. Provitamin A, better known as beta-carotene, is totally safe.

Recommended dosage: 10,000 I.U. as beta-carotene daily.

Omega-3 fatty acids. Some people with psoriasis have low levels of omega-3 fatty acids, which help nourish the skin.

Recommended dosage: 1 gram a day of fish oil containing EPA a day.

Flaxseed. Flaxseed, which helps restore normal oil production in the skin, contains omega-3 fatty acids.

Recommended dosage: 1 tablespoon of oil a day.

Oatmeal. An oatmeal bath can minimize itching associated with psoriasis. A handful in a tub of warm water should do the trick. Wrap the oatmeal in cheesecloth to prevent it from clogging the drain. Or use a commercial product sold as colloidal oatmeal.

WHEN TO CALL THE DOCTOR

If your skin erupts in large patches of dry, scaly skin, see a dermatologist for a diagnosis. Psoriasis can mimic symptoms of other skin disorders, such as eczema.

If you have psoriasis, have your skin routinely checked by a specialist. Psoriasis can sometimes lead to a more complicated skin disorder called seborrheic dermatitis, which involves a dysfunction of the skin's sebaceous glands. Only a dermatologist or other skin specialist can make an initial diagnosis and recommend a treatment plan.

RAYNAUD'S DISEASE

Cold hands, warm heart? If so, you could have Raynaud's disease, a mysterious condition that causes the blood vessels in the hands and feet to constrict and clamp down at the slightest sense of cold.

It can happen on a 100-degree day just by sticking your hand in the freezer to get ice cubes, or in the dead of winter, even if you're wearing double layers of socks and boots.

When the temperature drops, it is normal for blood vessels in the extremities to constrict. This is how your body conserves heat. For people with Raynaud's, however, this process is greatly exaggerated. It cuts off circulation to the point that hands and feet can turn from white to blue to red as circulation stops and restarts again. Attacks can last for minutes to hours.

Nobody knows what causes Raynaud's—otherwise perfectly healthy people can experience it. But it is also associated with circulatory conditions.

COLD CURES

Niacin. This form of vitamin B3 helps improve circulation.

Recommended dosage: 500 milligrams the form of inositol hexaniacinate three times a day with meals.

Ginkgo biloba. Dozens of studies show that ginkgo improves circulation but most of it focuses on blood flow to the brain. There is also evidence that it can improve blood flow in the extremities. In fact, European doctors commonly recommend ginkgo supplements to people with Raynaud's disease.

Recommended dosage: 40 to 80 milligrams of ginkgo biloba extract containing 24 percent flavone glycosides.

Pepper. According to folklore, people used to sprinkle cayenne pepper in their boots to keep their feet warm in winter. Aromatherapists recommend mixing it in a little oil and massaging it into the hands and feet. Black pepper works, too.

Garlic and onion. These herbs are well known for aiding circulation. Get them in your diet as much as possible. You can also try garlic supplements.

Recommended dosage: 800 milligrams a day.

Fish oil. There is some evidence that fish oil supplements can help ease the symptoms of Raynaud's.

Recommended dosage: 1,000 milligrams three times a day.

WHEN TO CALL THE DOCTOR

Raynaud's disease is not a serious condition. However, if you are experiencing the symptoms for the first time, discuss it with your doctor to rule out a circulation problem.

RESTLESS LEG SYNDROME

All you want to do is rest but your legs are ready to roam. They kick and jerk and just won't leave you alone. Restless leg syndrome could just as well be called restless sleep syndrome because its characteristic symptom keeps you awake at night.

Some people describe the feeling as a tingling, writhing, crawling sensation, or an itch deep inside the leg. It usually comes on when you're sitting in a chair and trying to relax, but it is most problematic at night. It can be so vexing that the only way for your body to respond is to get out of bed and walk.

Restless leg syndrome has only been recognized as a bona fide condition in recent years and there is no known cause or cure. There is a prescription medication to stop the restless feeling but it has some side effects that many people can't take. There are, however, a few natural alternatives.

LESS RESTLESS SOLUTIONS

Iron. Iron deficiency, due to an inability to properly absorb the mineral, has been associated with restless leg syndrome, especially in the elderly. A blood test can determine if you are low in iron.

Recommended dosage: 30 milligrams twice a day between meals.

Vitamin C. Vitamin C can enhance the absorption of iron.

Recommended dosage: 250 milligrams taken together with iron.

Magnesium. Research shows that magnesium supplementation can help ease restless legs.

Recommended dosage: 250 milligrams of magnesium citrate taken at bedtime.

Folic acid. Low levels of folate are also associated with restless leg syndrome, especially among those with a genetic predisposition to the condition.

Recommended dosage: 400 to 800 micrograms a day.

RHEUMATOID ARTHRITIS

Your immune system is your best defense. It protects you against harmful agents that try to attack your body and make you sick. Sometimes, though, your immune system can be the enemy, as is the case with rheumatoid arthritis.

Rheumatoid arthritis is a painful and debilitating disease in which the immune system turns on itself and attacks your joints and organs. It affects the entire body, causing chronic inflammation of many joints, as well as the skin, muscles, blood vessels, and in rare cases, organs such as the heart and lungs. It can even lead to joint deformity.

In addition to joint problems, rheumatoid arthritis can cause bouts of fever, fatigue, weight loss, anemia, and tingling hands and feet. If the organs become involved, complications can include an enlarged spleen, irregular heartbeat, or pleurisy, an inflammation of the membrane covering the lungs. Lumps, called rheumatoid nodules, can pop up in the joints, especially in the elbow joints.

THE ON-AND-OFF DISEASE

Once you get rheumatoid arthritis, it is with you for a lifetime, though the course of the disease is hard to predict. Some people experience a single bout and then the disease seems to disappear. (Doctors call this monocyclic rheumatoid arthritis.) For most people, though, painful cycles come and go. Most often, a diagnosis of rheumatoid arthritis means chronic pain and the need for pain management.

This serious condition plagues about seven million Americans, about three-fourths of them women. The first signs of the disease usually show up between the ages of 35 and 45.

The cause of rheumatoid arthritis is not fully understood, though heredity, food allergies, bacterial or viral infection, and the presence of certain antibodies in the blood all play a role. Management of the pain is ongoing, so natural therapy is often preferred to pharmaceutical solutions.

JOINT RELIEF

Fatty acids. Fish oils and omega-3 fatty acids have been shown to relieve inflammation and the symptoms of rheumatoid arthritis. A Danish study of 51 people with rheumatoid arthritis found significant improvement in stiffness and pain after 12 weeks on a daily dose of 3.6 grams of omega-3 polyunsaturated fatty acids. (The amount used in the study is equal to about one eight-ounce serving of salmon, mackerel, or herring.)

Recommended dosage: 1.2 milligrams of fish oil containing eicosapentaenoic acid (EPA) and 1.8 milligrams of docosahexaenoic acid (DHA) a day.

Selenium. Many people with rheumatoid arthritis have low levels of selenium, an important antioxidant that also helps slow the body's production of inflammatory agents known as prostaglandins and leukotrienes. Most good multivitamin–mineral supplements contain appropriate amounts of selenium (50 to 200 micrograms).

Vitamin B5. Pantothenic acid deficiency has been linked to rheumatoid arthritis. The lower the level of vitamin B5, the more severe the symptoms. Studies have found that raising vitamin B5 levels to the normal range helped alleviate symptoms. In one study, patients taking 2 grams of vitamin B5 experienced improvement in morning stiffness and pain.

Recommended dosage: Up to 2 grams of vitamin B5 daily.

Vitamin C. Without enough vitamin C, the body stops producing collagen, and the joints become compromised. Vitamin C also helps reduce inflammation associated with rheumatoid arthritis.

Recommended dosage: Up to 3,000 milligrams divided throughout the day.

Bromelain. The active ingredient in the pineapple plant helps the body get rid of immune antigen complex, compounds associated with rheumatoid arthritis.

Recommended dosage: 500 milligrams three times a day between meals.

Capsaicin. This is the active ingredient that makes cayenne pepper hot. In one study capsaicin cream helped reduce rheumatic joint pain by 50 percent. Apply the cream as directed.

WHEN TO CALL THE DOCTOR

Rheumatoid arthritis usually first shows up as pain when moving a joint, especially early in the morning. It usually occurs first in the wrists and knuckles, or the knee and ball of the foot, though it can affect any joint of the body. If you experience chronic or severe joint pain, consult with your doctor.

ROSACEA

You walk into the wind, and two minutes later you look like you're blushing even though you're not. The same thing happens when you sip a martini or eat spicy food. While a sudden blush doesn't seem like it should be a problem, it is if your blushing is caused by rosacea.

The problem with rosacea is that the blushing can become so persistent that it damages the blood vessels on the cheeks and nose. This can cause the redness to become more intense and the skin to become rough and thickened, giving the face a perpetual bumpy and sunburned appearance.

The cause of rosacea is unknown but there is evidence that it is involved with a faulty digestive system that causes the skin to excrete toxins that show up as a red, spotty face rash. Many people with rosacea have low levels of stomach acid that interrupts digestion and causes sluggish bowels.

STOP THE BLUSHING

Digestive enzymes. Lipase enzymes that help absorb fat are helpful to people with rosacea.

Recommended dosage: 1 or 2 capsules containing lipase a day.

Probiotics. Lactobacillus acidophilus and acidophilus bifidus are active organisms that supply the digestive system with friendly bacteria.

Recommended dosage: A product containing 4 billion active cultures twice a day between meals.

Betain Hydrochloride. This supplement increases stomach acidity and also helps improve digestion.

Recommended dosage: 1 to 3 capsules with meals.

B complex. A deficiency of B vitamins has been found in some people with rosacea.

Recommended dosage: 50 milligrams a day.

Vitamin B12. This vitamin has been found to reduce flare-ups of rosacea. For some people, however, it only works by injection. You should discuss it with your doctor if supplements don't help.

Recommended dosage: 400 to 800 micrograms.

Chamomile. The essential oil of chamomile is effective at reducing skin inflammation, but the oil can be reactive in a rash. Instead, steep several chamomile tea bags in a quart of hot water. Keep in the refrigerator or a cool place. Apply it with a soft cloth when you feel a flush coming on.

CARING FOR YOUR SKIN

Rosacea at times may resemble acne but there is no relationship between them. Acne treatments are not appropriate for rosacea and can even worsen flare-ups. Follow this advice.

- Cleanse your face with mild face soap. Buy soap for sensitive skin, such as Cetaphil, Aquanil, or Dove, that does not contain perfume or preservatives.
- Avoid any makeup or after-shave products containing alcohol, benzyl peroxide, menthol, salicylic acid, or witch hazel.
- Avoid alcohol, spicy foods, and sauna baths, which can all bring on an outbreak.
- Keep your face out of the sun and wear a nonabsorbing sunscreen, such as zinc oxide, when at the beach.

WHEN TO CALL THE DOCTOR

Do not try to self-diagnose rosacea. Because rosacea can damage blood vessel and cause other changes in the skin, you should consult with a dermatologist or skin care specialist for advice on the best ways to control the condition.

SEASONAL AFFECTIVE DISORDER

Come November, does your mood and interest in life take a nosedive and start back come April? If so, you may have Seasonal Affective Disorder, a depressionlike condition with an apropos acronym—SAD.

SAD is like a mental allergy to winter. As daylight hours get shorter with the approach and advance of the winter season, people with SAD are overcome with moodiness, depression, and lethargy. They tend to sleep more and eat more, especially sweets and other carbohydrates. Some people become antisocial, preferring to stay at home instead of going out. This can make SAD even worse.

While SAD is often considered one of those conditions that's "all in your head," scientists have found the decrease in daytime light can cause a change in brain chemistry. As exposure to light diminishes, the brain secretes the sleep-inducing hormone melatonin. In people with SAD, melatonin secretion is magnified. SAD affects an estimated 10 to 20 percent of people in the United States. It is more common in women than in men and is at its worst in January. People in the north, where temperatures are colder and winters are longer, are most affected.

EVEN MORE SAD

SAD isn't just a wintertime condition. Though less common, some people have a mental allergy to summer. And the symptoms are the opposite to winter SAD. They can't sleep, lose their appetites, and become restless. The higher the temperature and humidity, the more irritated they become.

A third type of SAD is also being investigated. It is a year-round SAD that affects people who work in a window-less environment.

LIGHT POWER

In addition to these remedies, you can follow the advice for depression on page 97.

Saint John's Wort. The flowers on this perennial shrub are as bright and yellow as sunshine. Its active ingredient, hypericin, is an effective natural antidepressant.

Recommended dosage: 300 milligrams a day.

SAMe. S-adenosyl-L-methionine is an amino acid that increases the brain chemicals that put you in a good mood.

Recommended dosage: 200 milligrams a day between meals.

B complex. B vitamins help the body metabolize SAMe.

Recommended dosage: 50 milligrams twice a day on an empty stomach.

Vitamin D. Studies show that the sunshine vitamin is a mood regulator. If you do not get into the sunshine every day, you should consider taking vitamin D.

Recommended dosage: Up to 1,000 I.U. daily.

Fish oil. Omega-3 fatty acids help improve neurotrans-mitter activity metabolism and activity in the brain.

Recommended dosage: A 500-milligram tablet contain-ing both EPA and DHA daily.

GET IN THE RIGHT HABITS

Get yourself outside. People with SAD tend to make excuses that keep them indoors. Don't do it. Exposure to natural light, even if it is a cloudy day, can help.

Let the light in. Open your home to natural light by keeping blinds and drapes open, even at night. Even if it is still dark when you wake up in the morning, you can get a lift when daylight comes streaming in through uncovered windowpanes.

Avoid alcohol. You've heard it before: alcohol may lift your spirits at first but the aftermath of drinking can make depression worse.

Balance your diet. Too many carbohydrates, especially the sweet variety, can affect your blood sugar, which affects your mood. Get protein with every meal and eat it first.

Take a winter vacation. If possible, plan a trip during the doldrums of winter. Even if you don't go someplace warm, the change of scenery will lift your spirits.

WHEN TO CALL THE DOCTOR

If the symptoms of SAD start interfering with your life, see a psychologist or an alternative therapist. There are some natural therapies, such as light treatments, that require a referral. One new treatment is a headband mounted with lights that delivers light to the retina. It allows you to go about your daily routine rather than sitting and doing nothing in a light box.

SINUSITIS

The sinuses are tiny holes in your head that act as your air-quality control center. These holes are actually empty spaces—one above and below each eye and two on each side of the nose—that are lined with membranes.

Mucus and tiny hairs called cilia are the stuff that stops dust particles from getting into the air that you breathe and keeps your breathing apparatus from getting dry and irritated.

When all is well, this system works well; mucus flows

freely in and out of your sinuses. But when the system gets gummed up—be it from a cold, an allergy, or some kind of infection—misery sets in. Your sinuses get clogged with gobs of mucus that reproduce faster than you can fill a tissue. Your head feels pumped with so much pressure it makes your eyes throb. It's bad during the day but gets worse at night when your prone position forces your sinuses to drip, drip down your throat, causing coughing spasms. It means you've got a ten-alarm sinus infection and it isn't pretty—for you or anyone who has to be around you, especially at night.

A COMMON PROBLEM

Like a cold, sinusitis is a common condition that strikes some 30 million people every year. It feels like a cold but only 10 times worse, and it lasts longer, too. For some people, though, sinusitis becomes a chronic problem. This is a warning that something else is going on that is wearing down your immune system.

Among the major suspects causing sinusitis are environmental allergens, such as cigarette smoke, environmental pollutants, mold spores, and fungus. It can also be caused by a dental infection, flying in an airplane, or other activities that put pressure on the sinuses. Hay fever can also turn into sinusitis.

NASAL PASSAGE OPENERS

Eucalyptus. The strong scent of eucalyptus can open nasal passages and make you breathe freely. Put a few drops of eucalyptus essential oil in the water of a facial steam. Aromatherapists suggest diluting it in a little oil and rubbing it on your forehead and next to your nasal passages.

Oregano and peppermint. If you don't care for the strong scent of eucalyptus, you can try the same with mint, which has powerful antiseptic qualities. (Oregano is a member of the mint family.)

Echinacea. This remarkable infection-fighter works best for sinusitis when taken as a tea and drunk throughout the day. Using the actual root rather than a commercial product will produce the best results. Use one teaspoon of cut and sifted echinacea root per cup of water. Bring to a boil and steep for 15 minutes. Strain into a container and drink, warmed up, throughout the day.

Garlic. Eating fresh garlic cloves reinforces healing by increasing the immune system's natural killer cell activity. If eating raw garlic doesn't appeal to you, take garlic tablets.

Recommended dosage: 10 milligrams a day until the infection is gone.

Turmeric. Its anti-inflammatory action helps reduce pressure on the sinuses.

Recommended dosage: 400 milligrams three times a day.

N-acetylcysteine. This nutrient helps thin mucus secretions so that the sinuses drain more effectively.

Recommended dosage: 500 milligrams four times a day.

Chicken soup. Grandma's home remedy is still one of the best therapies for any kind of respiratory infection. Make a pot of chicken soup loaded with fresh vegetables and lots of garlic.

Horseradish. For a quick route to easy breathing, take a deep sniff from a bottle of strong horseradish. Or, if you can take it, heap horseradish on a piece of bread and eat it. Doing this before bedtime will help keep sinus passages free during the night.

WHEN TO CALL THE DOCTOR

If self-treatment doesn't improve your sinus condition after a few days or the problem gets worse instead of better, call your doctor. Though rare, sinusitis can lead to pneumonia or even meningitis.

SORE THROAT

You know you're in for a rough day when you wake up in the morning with a throat so scratchy and sore that it is painful to swallow.

If you didn't spend the night before exercising your vocal cords to excess at a loud event like a rock concert or bowl game, it means that you're headed for a cold, flu, or some kind of viral infection. Chances are, if you let yourself fall back to sleep, you'll awaken in a few hours with a stuffy nose and possibly a fever and the chills. Don't hide your head under the pillow! If you take action fast you might be able to beat down whatever it is that's trying to sneak up on you.

THROAT SOOTHERS

Saltwater plus. Warm salted water is an excellent gargle to soothe a sore throat but for a really effective remedy add some lemon juice, apple cider vinegar, and a teaspoon of honey. Gargle every hour.

Horehound. Tea feels good on a sore throat, so get some extra healing action by brewing two teaspoons of chopped herb for every cup of water. Horehound helps reduce swelling in the throat. Drink throughout the day.

Echinacea. You can turn a cold away at the pass if you get it early enough with this well-known viral fighter. *Recommended dosage:* 200 milligrams with standardized 3.5% echinacosides.

Vitamin C. Start dosing with vitamin C to reinforce your immune system.

Recommended dosage: 1,000 milligrams taken throughout the day.

HYDROTHERAPY THE DAY

You'll want to get plenty of liquids in you. Drink fruit juices for extra vitamin fortification in addition to drinking plenty of water. Here are a few other things you can do.

- Heat a neck wrap (follow manufacturer's directions) and snuggle with it for 15 minutes every few hours.
- Add moisture to your immediate environment with a cool-mist vaporizer or humidifier. Or, heat a pot of water and add a few drops of essential oil, such as echinacea or astragalus, and take a few whiffs of the pot. Be careful not to get too close.
- Mix up a batch of chicken soup containing lots of garlic and vegetables. It will not only feel good on your throat but will help fight infection.

WHEN TO CALL THE DOCTOR

A sore throat is not something to ignore, especially if the pain increases and you feel like you are coming down with something worse than a cold or the flu. It is possible you could have strep throat.

Strep throat is a bacterial infection that needs to be treated with antibiotics. Strep is a serious problem because, left untreated, it can lead to rheumatic fever and rheumatic heart disease, which damages the heart valve. If you have any of these symptoms, seek medical help.

- Swollen glands
- Earache
- Rash or fever above 101
- Blood in saliva or phlegm

STRESS

Stress is an important and natural part of life, and a certain amount is healing and positive. It can keep us motivated, lift our spirits, and bring us joy.

The stress associated with being in love, learning how to drive, or playing in a big game are typically thought of as positive stress. But in today's fast-paced society, we are surrounded by more negative stress than ever before. From sitting in traffic jams to answering e-mail and cell phones at the same time, to keeping the kids busy and the household going, to caring for aging parents, to new toasters that require owners manuals to operate. Living may be easier than ever but at the same time it is a lot more complicated!

Then there are environmental stressors, such as air pollution, noise pollution, food chemicals, alcohol, caffeine, and nicotine, as well as emotional stressors, such as feelings of guilt, fear, and sorrow.

All of this can accumulate and leave us feeling pretty strung out and on the verge of crumbling into a big ball of confusion.

BACKLASH TO HEALTH

The human body is equipped with a system of checks and balances to deal with stress. During a stressful situation, the sympathetic nervous system, which is part of the central nervous system, sends the hormones adrenaline and noradrenaline into the bloodstream. This raises heart rate, breathing rate, and blood pressure. It makes you feel tense.

In an effort to relieve this feeling, the parasympathetic nervous system secretes a hormone called acetylcholine, which can reduce heart rate and improve digestion. When you continue to feel stressed, however, the parasympathetic nervous system can't do its job well, and your body tries to adapt to your higher level of stress.

When you're under stress, your adrenal glands over-secrete hormones, which can interfere with the function of the immune system cells that are responsible for warding off infection. This eventually drains the body and throws it out of balance, creating nutritional deficiencies, and a host of stress symptoms, including fatigue, headaches, and susceptibility to illnesses.

Each individual responds to stress in a different way and to different degrees but we all can benefit from learning how to manage stress.

ANTI-STRESS SOLUTIONS

Chamomile. This aromatic herb can bring on calm when you most need it. Buy a bottle of essential oil and put it in a lamp ring next to a comfortable chair to help you relax. Buy the dried flowers and brew it into a tea that you can sip throughout the day. During tense moments, put a few drops on a tissue, put your nose up close, and breathe in deeply.

Valerian. This herb contains compounds that help induce calm. If you are chronically stressed, valerian will help ease stress-induced mental tension.

Recommended dosage: 150 milligrams twice a day.

Kava kava. This stress reducer works by helping to ease wound-up muscles brought on by stress and physical tension.

Recommended dosage: 200 milligrams three times a day.

Lavender. This is another aromatic herb that promotes relaxation. Buy a vial of lavender oil and breathe from it as recommended above for chamomile. Put a few drops in a bath at night to help you relax and fall asleep.

LEARNING TO RELAX

Meditation. Research shows that regular meditation reduces stress hormones, slows breathing rate, and increases alpha brain waves, which are associated with relaxation. There are many ways to meditate, including learning the discipline of transcendental meditation.

Deep breathing. As babies we breathe properly—through the abdomen, which maximizes oxygen intake and stimulates every cell in the body. As we grow up, however, we somehow get out of this habit and start breathing from the chest, which is less efficient. Belly breathing can go a long way in helping to relieve stress. If you can get in the habit of belly breathing, at least pause several times a day to take a long, deep breath.

Take time for yourself. Women, especially, are guilty of doing all for others and taking no time for themselves. Studies show that this can produce the kind of stress that leads to heart disease.

Yoga. Exercise in general is a well-studied antidote to stress. In addition to your routine exercise, learn a few yoga poses to help you relax, especially at bedtime.

Eat well. Stay away from saturated fats and eat high-energy foods, such as nuts and whole grains. Avoid caffeine, alcohol, and complete your diet with whole grains, fruits, and vegetables.

SUNBURN

How can something so good for you also be so bad? After all, life wouldn't exist without the sun.

The sun *is* good for you, as long as you take it as you should everything in life—in moderation. And moderation in the sun is considered 15 minutes a day of early morning or late afternoon *sunlight*—not bronzing on the beach at high noon in the middle of summer.

Everyone knows the hazards of the sun. It accelerates aging and promotes skin cancer. It can also lead to cataracts. Nevertheless, a day on the beach is hard to resist and sometimes, even when you have the best intentions and wear sunscreen, sunglasses and a hat, you can end up scorched by the sun. Here's what to do when it happens.

GETTING THE RED OUT

Cucumber. There is merit in the expression, *cool as a cucumber*. A fresh cold cucumber can take the sting and pain out of sunburn. Just slice it and lay it over your skin for 10 or 15 minutes. Wrap a towel around it if necessary to hold the cucumber in place.

Aloe. The gel from the aloe vera plant is proven to speed the healing of minor burns. Buy it as a commercial cream or keep a plant handy on the windowsill. Just snip and squeeze the gel onto your sun-exposed skin.

Prickly pear. The gel inside the leaf of this cactus plant works the same as aloe. Cut a leaf in half and press it against the skin. You can find prickly pear in the vegetable sections of many supermarkets.

Black tea. Tea contains astringent tannins that can soothe sun-sore skin. Take the tea, let it cool and refrigerate. Dab it on your skin with a soft cloth.

Vitamin E. This oily nutrient is often recommended for skin problems, including sunburn. By a sunburn cream containing vitamin E or open a vitamin E capsule and rub it into the burn.

L-selenomethionine. Studies show that this amino acid

can reduce the damage caused by sunburn. You can apply it to the skin or take it orally.

Recommended dosage: 100 micrograms a day.

PAY ATTENTION TO PREVENTION

Sunscreen. Sunscreen. Sunscreen. Make it a habit, not just when you are going to the beach but on a daily basis, especially if you live in areas of the country where the sun is the strongest, such as Arizona.

Apply a sunscreen with a sun protection factor (SPF) of at least 15. SPF refers to the amount of time you can expose your skin to the sun without burning. For example, if your unexposed skin would start to burn in 10 minutes, then a sunscreen with a SPF of 15 will keep you safe in the sun 15 times longer, or 150 minutes. Also, look for makeup that contains sunscreen.

TOOTHACHE

A toothache is one of the few things that can get someone begging to see a dentist.

A toothache can be searing, life-suspending pain. And for some reason with no scientific explanation, they tend to occur at the most inopportune times—like a Friday or Saturday night when relief is *two days away.* But you can at least find temporary relief just a few steps away—in your kitchen.

NUMBING SOLUTIONS

Clove. The cloves that you use to spike your holiday ham contain an oily substance called eugenol that acts as a super local anesthetic. In fact, back in the days when dentistry was pure torture, dentists used oil of clove to help ease the pain of dental procedures.

If you don't have oil of clove handy in your medicine chest, just pop a few cloves in your mouth, moisten them with your saliva, and let them release their oil against your painful tooth. Leave them for about 30 minutes, then spit them out.

Cayenne. Red pepper can also produce a numbing effect. Put a few tablespoons in a shallow dish and add just enough water to make a paste. Saturate a cotton ball with the paste and hold it against the painful tooth. Cayenne contains capsaicin, which has the ability to stop the action of substance P, the chemical responsible for transmitting the sensation of pain.

Ginger. Powdered ginger is a counterirritant that has an effect on toothache similar to cayenne. Mix and apply it the same way.

Rhubarb. The root of the rhubarb plant contains at least six compounds with pain-relieving action. Fry the root, then steep it in alcohol to make a tincture. Saturate a cotton ball in the substance and apply it to the pained tooth.

Sesame. Boil one part sesame seeds in two parts of water. Let it cool until warm and swish it around your sore tooth. Sesame contains several pain-relieving compounds.

WHEN TO CALL THE DOCTOR

A toothache is a siren that something is awry in your dental health. Even if the toothache goes away, make an appointment with your dentist.

ULCERS

Anyone can get an ulcer—and about one in every 10 Americans does.

Ulcers form when powerful digestive juices start to burn

through the delicate lining of the gastrointestinal tract, causing open lesions or sores. As you can imagine, this causes a certain amount of pain, much like a burning or gnawing sensation, in the upper abdomen.

Ulcers form for one of two reasons: you have too much stomach acid, or you have a weakness in the mucous lining that protects the digestive tract.

There are two kinds of ulcers: gastric, which appear in the stomach, and duodenal, which form in the duodenum (the first part of the small intestine). Duodenal ulcers are about five times more common than gastric ulcers and about four times more common in men than in women.

THE BACTERIAL CONNECTION

Long gone are the days when ulcers were associated with the overworked, hard-living man with a wife and a bunch of kids to support. While stress might play a part in causing an ulcer, this is not the real cause. Researchers have found that many ulcers are caused or exacerbated by a bacterium known as *Helicobacter pylori*. Research shows that the bacterium is present in up to 100 percent of patients with duodenal ulcer and in up to 70 percent of those with gastric ulcer. Factors that predispose to infection by *H. pylori* include low levels of antioxidants in the stomach and intestinal linings and low gastric acid production. A two-week regimen of antibiotics can wipe out this bacterium, vastly diminishing the odds of a recurrence. People who take large doses of stomach-irritating, anti-inflammatory drugs to manage pain are at increased risk of developing ulcers. They also tend to run in families.

The gnawing cramplike pain that is a warning sign of an ulcer usually comes on forty-five to sixty minutes after eating or during the night. This distress is relieved by food, antacids, or vomiting.

Though you should be under a doctor's care for an ulcer, there are things you can do on your own to manage the problem.

TAMING A TENDER TUMMY

Ginger. When you feel your ulcer acting up, pop a piece of candied ginger in your mouth. The same properties that come to the aid of a queasy stomach can also help soothe a stomach ulcer.

Chamomile. German herbalists highly rate chamomile for an ulcer because of its stomach-soothing properties. Drink it as a tea throughout the day.

Licorice. Deglycyrrhizinated licorice, or DLG, is an extract of the licorice herb that contains anti-ulcer compounds. A three-month study found DGL worked better than the popular drug, Tagamet, in helping people with duodenal ulcers. Commercially prepared DGL products are available; follow package directions.

Recommended dosage: 500 milligrams three times a day before meals.

Aloe vera. The juice of the aloe vera plant helps heal the lining of the stomach. Drink about an ounce a day or use a supplement.

Recommended dosage: 50 to 200 milligrams of powder or as a powdered capsule a day.

Vitamin C. This antioxidant has been found to retard the growth of *H. pylori*. It also helps protect the stomach lining.

Recommended dosage: 500 milligrams three times daily.

Cabbage juice. The juice squeezed from raw cabbage offers concentrated amounts of glutamine and S-methylmethionine, two compounds with anti-ulcer activity.

Banana. If you can't handle drinking cabbage juice daily, try eating a banana. There is some scientific validity to the old wives' tale that banana can soothe an ulcer.

Psyllium. Fiber is associated with a reduced rate of duodenal ulcer; it also cuts recurrence rates of the illness. Fiber promotes the secretion of mucus, which helps protect the digestive tract. Psyllium is a natural fiber. Begin with half a teaspoon of psyllium seeds or powder mixed in 8 ounces of cool liquid and drink 2 to 3 cups daily. Stir the mixture vigorously and drink it quickly, followed by additional water.

PAY ATTENTION TO PREVENTION

Food can help neutralize stomach acid, so don't go too long without eating. Eat six small meals a day rather than three larger ones. You can also minimize your risk of getting an ulcer by following this advice.

- Eliminate alcohol.
- Minimize your intake of caffeine.
- Quit smoking. Tobacco smoke constricts the blood vessels lining the stomach, making the stomach wall more vulnerable to sores.
- Avoid the use of aspirin and other nonsteroidal antiinflammatory drugs, which are associated with the formation of ulcers.

WHEN TO CALL THE DOCTOR

Left untreated, an ulcer can lead to serious illness, such as peritonitis, an inflammation of the lining of the abdominal cavity. In severe cases, an ulcer can burn a hole right through the stomach or intestine. This is called a perforated ulcer and is considered a medical emergency.

Signs of a bleeding ulcer include vomiting blood or

material that looks like coffee grounds, and passing black, tar-like stools. Call your doctor right away.

URINARY TRACT INFECTIONS

When just the thought of having to go to the bathroom makes you wince, you know you have a urinary tract infection, or what veterans of the infection call a UTI.

Burning during urination is the telltale sign of a UTI. To make matters worse, a UTI tends to make you want to urinate a lot.

The problem with getting one UTI is that you're likely to get another, and another. Urinary tract infections are quite common and many people, particularly women, are susceptible to them.

THREE KINDS OF TROUBLE

Bacteria that originate in the intestine and reside quite harmlessly in the area around the anus cause more than 80 percent of UTIs. Trouble begins when they migrate into the urethra. Sex or clumsiness while handling tissue paper when you're on the toilet are two common ways this can happen. UTIs are more common in women because the trip from the anus to the urethra is a lot shorter than it is in a man.

The urinary system is interconnected so infection tends to spread. Depending on its directional course, UTIs come in three common types: *urethritis,* an infection of the tube that leads from the bladder to the outside of the body; *cystitis,* infection of the bladder; and *pyelitis,* an infection of the kidneys. The condition should be treated at the first sign of problems.

The common course of treatment for a UTI is antibiotics. There are some natural medicines that can work just as well or in concert with medication.

BLADDER PROTECTORS

Echinacea. Take this immune-boosting herb to help enhance the effects of antibiotics. Take one or two drops a day or as a capsule.

Recommended dosage: 500 milligrams a day.

Goldenseal. Herbalists consider goldenseal a natural antibiotic. It is also protective against bacteria adhering to the intestinal wall.

Recommended dosage: 250 to 500 milligrams of standardized root a day.

Uva ursi. The active ingredient in this herb, arbutin, acts as an antibacterial agent. It also acts as a diuretic.

Recommended dosage: 250 milligrams as arbutin in capsule form a day.

Vitamin C. This immune-enhancing vitamin acidifies urine, which helps eliminate the bacteria. *Note:* If you are also taking an antibiotic, check with your physician before taking vitamin C, as it may interfere with the effectiveness of the antibiotic.

Recommended dosage: 1,500 or 3,000 milligrams divided throughout the day.

Acidophilus. This "friendly bacteria" help restore the population of "good" bacteria in the intestinal tract.

Recommended dosage: 2 capsules three times daily.

Cranberry. Drinking cranberry juice is a well-known preventative for a bladder infection but it can also help speed the healing action. If you have an active infection you might want to try cranberry extract.

Recommended dosage: 400 milligrams twice a day.

PAY ATTENTION TO PREVENTION

You can help prevent future infections by fortifying your immune system with antioxidant foods and supplements. You can also be more diligent about your bathroom hygiene.

For women, this means wiping from front to back after bowel movements to avoid fecal contamination of the urethra. Also, use white, unscented toilet paper and mild soaps when bathing.

WHEN TO CALL THE DOCTOR

A UTI can sometimes turn into something more serious, such as bladder disease. Other conditions can also mimic symptoms of a UTI. Call your doctor if you experience any of these symptoms along with painful urination.

- Blood in the urine
- Pain in the lower back
- Fever
- Nausea or vomiting

VARICOSE VEINS

Varicose veins could just as well be called very close veins considering all the attention they draw—and the great lengths many people go to hide them.

More than 40 million Americans live with the swollen and sometimes painful veins that protrude like major intersections of blue byways snaking under the skin of ankles, calves, and thighs.

Gravity is to blame for the formation of varicose veins. Blood that circulates to the legs must be pumped uphill to the heart, against the pull of gravity. Veins are equipped with one-way valves to prevent the blood from flowing back down the legs, but when the valves are stretched or damaged, they don't close properly, and the blood slips back down and pools, causing the veins to stretch out and appear blue and puffy.

FEMALE FRIENDLY

Women experience varicose veins about four times more often than men, partially because of the rigor of pregnancy and childbirth. In preparation for childbirth a pregnant woman's body releases hormones that weaken the collagen and connective tissues in the pelvis to make the birth process easier. But these hormones can also weaken the collagen and valves in the veins, increasing the likelihood of varicose veins.

Other common causes of varicose veins include standing for long periods (the pressure exerted against the veins can increase up to ten times when standing), and sitting for long periods without movement, especially with the legs crossed. Genetics and obesity also contribute to the problem.

Bilberry. Anthocyanosides, the pigment that gives bilberry its vivid color, helps support the circulatory system. Bilberry strengthens vein walls and connective tissue.

Recommended dosage: 80 milligrams of extract standardized to 25% anthocyanosides three times a day.

Butcher's broom. Two compounds in this herb, ruscogenin and neoruscogenin, help constrict and strengthen veins.

Recommended dosage: 200 to 300 milligrams a day.

Witch hazel. Manufactured as an alcohol-based extract, witch hazel can be used externally to help strengthen vein walls.

Essential oils. Ease the pain and tension on varicose veins with a massage oil spiked with a few drops of the essential oils cypress, lavender, or bergamot.

Psyllium. This natural fiber can be used to build bulk in the stool and reduce straining during bowel movements. Over time, the straining of constipation can weaken the vein walls, resulting in varicose veins or hemorrhoids (varicose veins in the anus). Use a commercially prepared product and follow package directions.

Vitamin C. This antioxidant promotes healthy veins and circulation and reduces the risk of potentially dangerous blood clots from forming in the legs.

Recommended dosage: 1,000 milligrams taken throughout the day.

PAY ATTENTION TO PREVENTION

If varicose veins run in your family you should avoid habits that are hard on your veins. You can reduce your risk of getting varicose veins.

- Avoid standing for long periods of time, crossing your legs, lifting heavy objects, and wearing tight shoes, garters, or undergarments.
- Get regular exercise, especially walking, biking, and jogging. The contraction of the leg muscles helps move the pooled blood in the legs back into circulation.

WHEN TO CALL THE DOCTOR

Varicose veins that can be seen near the surface of the skin may appear sinister but generally they do not pose a health risk. Varicose veins, however, can form beneath the skin. This is the type that can cause serious and sometimes even life-threatening complications, such as skin ulcers, phlebitis (inflammation of the vein), and thrombosis (formation of a blood clot). These conditions require immediate medical attention.

If you experience sharp leg pans or notice a red lump in the vein that doesn't go away when you put your legs up, contact your doctor immediately.

VERTIGO

When the world is spinning around you but you're standing still, you have vertigo.

Vertigo is often mislabeled as the fear of heights (acrophobia), but it is the medical term for dizziness. It can sometimes last for a few seconds or minutes, like when you step off a boat and feel disoriented or when you get off a roller coaster and feel nauseated. In its most extreme form, vertigo can be totally debilitating, leaving you unable to stand without falling or open your eyes without seeing your line of vision spin wildly. The slightest move can cause vomiting.

Vertigo is not a condition; rather it is a symptom of something else affecting the inner ear, the balance center of the body. Any number of things can be the root of the problem, from something as minor as a buildup of earwax to a serious neurological disorder. It is possible that the source may never be found. For some people, vertigo can come, disappear for years, and suddenly reappear for no apparent reason.

SPIN DOCTORING

Ginger. Vertigo is motion sickness of the worse kind, so it goes without reason that what is helpful for one can help the other. Drink it daily as a tea or take supplements.

Recommended dosage: 300 to 500 milligrams a day.

Ginkgo. One study of people with chronic vertigo found a significant improvement in the symptom after taking ginkgo.

Recommended dosage: 60 to 240 milligrams a day.

Lavender. This essential oil can help bring calm and

stability when you are weak in the knees. Carry a vial with you and take a whiff whenever you start to feel woozy.

WHEN TO CALL THE DOCTOR

If you are getting dizzy spells, you should see a doctor for a thorough examination to help get to the source of the problem.

WARTS

You don't have to touch a toad to get a wart, and you don't have to see a doctor to get rid of one.

You may *think* that you need a doctor when you learn that a wart is really a skin tumor and it is caused by a virus with a serious-sounding name—human papillomavirus, also known as HPV. But the tumor is benign and the virus is as common as a virus can get.

Don't be concerned if you have a cluster of warts instead of a single wart. This is common, too. Warts, by the way, usually show up on the hand but can appear on other parts of the body. (A wart on the foot is called a plantar wart.)

Standard medical treatment often comes in the form of nasty-sounding destructive techniques that involve burning, scraping, freezing, injecting, or zapping with a laser. These may or may not be effective. Or you can just as easily try one of the many folk remedies for warts that have stood the test of time.

WART WARFARE

Birch bark. This herb contains two substances with antiviral activity: betulin and betulinic acid. It also contains salicylates, which the Food and Drug Administration has approved for treatment of warts. If you happen to have a birch tree in your yard, pick up a piece of fallen bark, moisten it and secure it, inner side directly on top of the wart, with tape. Keep it on until the bark dries. Repeat with fresh bark until the wart disappears. Or, brew a tea made with powdered birch bark and rub it on the wart.

Willow. You can do the same with the bark of the willow tree as you would with the bark of a birch tree. Or look for an over-the-counter wart preparation containing willow, which also goes by the name *Salix*.

Bloodroot. Look for a lotion containing bloodroot. The herb contains enzymes that help dissolve warts.

Dandelion. Rub the wart with the milky substance that oozes when you break the root of the dandelion plant. Apply it several times a day.

Lemon. The pith, or inside white part, of a lemon contains oil with potent antiseptic properties. Tape a piece of lemon to the wart when you go to bed at night. Or mix a few drops of lemon essential oil into an unscented lotion and rub it into the wart.

Vitamin C. The acidic nature of vitamin C can be highly effective against warts. Grind up a few vitamin C tablets and mix with just enough water to make a paste. Rub it into the wart and cover it with a bandage.

WHEN TO CALL THE DOCTOR

Warts are nothing to be concerned about. In fact, the only reason to get rid of a wart is if it is unslightly or it causes irritation as a result of getting in the way of routine living. Keep in mind, however, that warts can hang around for a long time—even for a year or two.

Also, make sure that what has popped up on your skin is actually a wart. Warts look like pale, skin-colored bumps on the surface of the skin with a rough surface and smooth borders. If in doubt, have the diagnosis made by a doctor.

WRINKLES

They say that age is defined by how well you feel, not by how good you look. However, if you're a 40-year-old who feels like a 15-year-old but looks more like a 50-year-old, it can be hard to find the wisdom in these words.

Sure, there are a lot of good things that go along with getting older—wisdom, independence, and a seat at the bar, to name but a few—but wrinkles on the face and sagging arms and thighs are definitely not among them.

Actually, the aging process begins almost at the moment of birth when the skin is cleansed of fluid and exposed to air.

THE LINES OF TIME

The skin starts to look old as a result of a lifetime of exposure to the elements. This is due to oxidation, a chemical process that causes anything—be it an Adirondack chair or your skin—to show wear and tear. Consider how tough the weather is on an outdoor chair. If you don't season the wood and protect it with paint or varnish, it's going to dry out and show wear before its time. The same can be said for the skin.

About 70 percent of the skin is made up of collagen, connective tissue that is mostly elastic. Collagen maintains its elasticity and smooth appearance by absorbing moisture. Sebum provides the internal "seasoning" that keeps collagen lubricated.

Oxidation can't be avoided. It is a natural part of the aging process in which highly reactive molecules called free radicals continually bombard the body and try to wear it down. The body, however, has its own built-in defense mechanism known as the immune system, which protects all the body's organs and keeps them healthy and strong by fighting off free radicals. The largest organ in the body—the skin—is the only organ that is directly exposed to the elements, so it takes a lot of abuse. By about age 30, the wear and tear starts to show in the form of fine lines around the eyes. This is when the production of sebum starts to slow and collagen begins to break down.

How rapidly this happens and the age at which it actually begins to show depends largely on the abuse the skin has taken by the elements. The skin's biggest enemies are the sun, environmental toxins, and nicotine, which attract free radicals as if the skin were fly paper. Emotional stress can wear on the skin just like it wears on the heart. Repeatedly gaining and losing weight can overtax the elasticity of collagen and cause it to break down faster. A diet deficient in free-radical fighting antioxidants, lack of sleep, and living in an arid climate can also cause premature aging.

It takes time to develop wrinkles, and you can't get rid of them overnight. In fact, unless you submit yourself to cosmetic surgery, you'll never really get rid of them. And even then, the process only starts all over again.

The true secret to youthful skin is a lifetime habit of nourishing your skin with the proper nutrients—both internally and externally—and avoiding exposure to skin-damaging ultraviolet light. But you can help diminish the lines of time and protect the skin against present and future abuse with a regimen of skin-nurturing natural substances and lifestyle practices.

SKIN-SAVING SOLUTIONS

Moisturizers containing any of these agents are helpful for skin that is already showing signs of aging. Keep in mind that using anything that contains antioxidants, especially vitamin C, will make your skin more vulnerable to the sun. So you should avoid the sun as much as possible and always wear sunscreen.

Antioxidant vitamins. It only makes sense that a smart way to fight oxidation is with antioxidants. Vitamin A is an antioxidant that gets high marks as a skin saver because it contains retinol, which stimulates skin cell renewal. Look for topical creams that contain the vitamin A retinoid analogs tretinoin and tazarotene. Also, make sure your diet contains plenty of antioxidant vegetables and fruits, especially those that contain vitamin A. Shoot for nine servings a day.

Vitamin C esters. This is vitamin-C-containing fatty acids, which helps the skin absorb antioxidants deeper and more rapidly than vitamin C alone. Vitamin C is essential to maintaining the elasticity of collagen. Vitamin C also helps another antioxidant, vitamin E, regenerate new skin. Studies show that topical vitamin C creams can help fight sun-damaged skin. Common wisdom says this is why lemon and lime wedges in drinking water put an extra kick in nourishing your skin.

Alpha-hydroxy acids. Also look for alpha-hydroxy acids, or AHAs, on the list of ingredients in moisturizing cream. Concentrated AHAs, which are derived from vitamin C, encourage collagen growth.

DHEA. The anti-aging activity of the hormone dehydroepiandrosterone is mostly focused on its ability to improve memory and sexual performance but it has skin-protective effects as well. According to studies on mice, topical DHEA is an antioxidant defense against the harmful rays of the sun and other everyday insults to the skin caused by pollutants in air, food, and water.

DMAE. Dimethylamineothanol is another substance produced in the brain that has anti-aging characteristics. Preliminary research shows that DMAE, when used as a topical agent, can help strengthen weakening elasticity of collagen.

Cocoa. Look on a bottle of moisturing cream and chances are that you'll see cocoa butter in the list of ingredients. It helps put moisture back in the skin and make it look plumper. It is especially good for the fine lines around the eyes.

Papaya. This tropical fruit contains proteolytic enzymes, which can act as a natural chemical peel. Herbalists mix mashed papaya with dry oatmeal and apply it to the face to remove dead and dry skin.

Avocado and olive oils. The oils in both avocado and olive oils are emollients that will help plump up the skin. Look for lotions that contain either of these oils.

BABY YOUR SKIN

Water. Picture a fresh plum next to a dried plum and it's easy to understand how important water is to the skin. Sip on water throughout the day and make sure to get at least 8 glasses.

Exercise. In addition to all the good exercise does for your mind, body, and spirit, sweating helps moisturize your skin. Just make sure to replace the fluids lost during exercising.

Sleep. When you don't sleep well at night, the next day you will look as dragged-out as you feel. Your skin is like the rest of your body—it does its replenishing while you are asleep.

This replenishing act, however, doesn't seem so obvious when you look in the mirror first thing in the morning and see lines across your face. These sleep lines are caused by sleeping on your side or stomach and snuggling your face deep in your pillow. The older you get, the longer it takes for sleep lines to fade. You can help avoid them by sleeping on a satin pillow case.

Eat well. Processed foods are loaded with chemicals, which contribute to toxic buildup. Avoid them and opt for a totally natural diet that includes lots and lots of fruits and vegetables.

The sun. Sun damage is the leading cause of premature aging. So forget the suntan. Enjoy the sun under the brim of a hat and behind a pair of sunglasses. Make sure to always wear sunscreen.

YEAST INFECTIONS

Spend the entire day and half the night standing, sitting, and walking around in tight leather pants and even tighter control-top panties and it's no surprise that you can't wait to crawl out of them at night. Don't be surprised, however, if you also feel like you want to crawl out of your skin.

Tight clothes that trap heat and moisture prevent ventilation, making the genital area a breeding ground for *candida albicans*, a vaginal yeast infection that causes itching, burning, and a thick, off-smelling discharge.

A COMMON NUISANCE

Candida is actually no stranger to a woman's body. It is present in minute amounts in the vagina but is kept in check by friendly bacteria in the body called lactobacilli. *Candida* is also kept in check by the immune system. Trouble starts to brew, however, when this well-balanced vaginal system is set off balance.

In addition to tight clothing, other circumstances that can upset the vaginal environment include chemical douches, deodorized mini pads, perfumed bathroom tissue, and even sex.

Yeast infections are quite common. An estimated one in four women will experience at least one yeast infection.

OUT WITH THE YEAST

Probiotics. The live cultures *lactobacillus acidophilus* and *lactobacillus bifidus* can correct the vaginal environment. Eating yogurt is helpful in preventing infections, but if you are in the throes of a bout you should opt for tablets.

Recommended dosage: 4 billion active organisms twice a day.

Garlic. Garlic is a potent fungus fighter. Again, the herb is a helpful preventative but try garlic capsules to get rid of infection.

Recommended dosage: 500 milligrams tablets twice a day.

Cranberry. Arbutin, a compound found in cranberries, has been found to help clear up yeast infections. Drink it freely until the infection clears up.

Echinacea. This powerful immune-enhancing herb stimulates white blood cells that gobble up yeast organisms.

White vinegar. Douching is generally not recommended because it can cause yeast infections. However, when in the throes of a yeast infection a vinegar douche may be just what you need. Add 2 tablespoons of white vinegar to a quart of warm water and douche twice a day for two days.

Sea salt. Take a warm-water bath containing a cup of dissolved sea salt. It will help ease the itching.

Sugar. Yeast feeds on glucose, so avoid sugary foods until you get rid of the infection. This includes white bread, honey, molasses, pasta, and alcohol.

PAY ATTENTION TO PREVENTION

Avoid scents. Fragrances used in tampons, toilet tissue, and female hygiene products can upset the delicate vaginal environment.

Wear breathable clothes. Avoid tight clothing and wearing pantyhose under form-fitting slacks. Also avoid sitting around in a wet bathing suit. Also, shed the underwear under your nightgown or pajamas.

WHEN TO CALL THE DOCTOR

If you've never before been diagnosed with a yeast infection you should see your doctor to confirm the diagnosis. You should also consult your doctor if you are pregnant or have diabetes and contract a yeast infection.

APPENDIX A
FOOD AS MEDICINE

EVERY TIME YOU put food in your mouth, you are making a choice that your body has to live with. A healthy diet—that is, one devoid of processed foods and as low as you can go in saturated fat—is essential to your overall health and well-being. In the last several decades, however, scientists have found that there is an abundance of nutrients with the ability to do more than support good health—they also have the power to help prevent and, even in some instances, help cure disease. This book offers many recommendations for taking nutritional supplements for more than 85 common health conditions. In some instances, specific foods are recommended. If your body is deficient or in need of extra stores of a certain nutrient, get familiar will the nutrient's best food choices and incorporate them into your diet. Following you will find healthy food choices for the nutrients listed in this book.

CALCIUM

Dairy products are best known as excellent calcium choices but here's a fact that may surprise you: low-fat versions contain more calcium than full-fat versions. Foods to go for include these.

Buttermilk
Carob
Cocoa
Gruyère cheese
Low-fat and nonfat yogurt
Low-fat and skim milk
Monterey Jack cheese
Part-skim ricotta cheese
Spinach
Swiss cheese

CAROTENES

More than 500 kinds of carotenes have been discovered, the most common being beta-carotene. Dark green and orange pigments in fruits and vegetables indicate the presence of carotene. These are among the best.

Bell peppers
Carrots
Collards
Kale
Papaya
Pumpkin
Spinach
Sweet potatoes
Tomatoes
Winter squash

COPPER

Copper is found in organ meats, which you want to avoid because of their super-high cholesterol count. Instead, go for these.

Chicken breast
Collard greens

Eggs
Endive
Kale
Legumes
Nuts
Peas

FIBER

You want to incorporate both soluble and insoluble fiber into your diet. Soluble fiber, meaning it dissolves in water, helps regulate blood sugar and also helps lower cholesterol. Insoluble fiber is the indigestible variety that helps support good digestive and bowel health. You should get 25 grams of total fiber a day.

Soluble fiber

Apples
Articokes
Beans
Blackberries
Blueberries
Lentils
Oat bran
Raisins

Insoluble Fiber

Apples
Artichokes
Banana
Blackberries
Broccoli
Brussels sprouts
Nuts
Peaches

Peas
Wheat bran

FOLATE

Organ meats are among the best source of folate but their sky-high cholesterol count does not make them a good choice for obvious reason. The smart solution is to go for the best source in the plant world. A serving of most types of beans will give you close to 50 percent of the DV.

Asparagus
Beans (adzuki, black, kidney, navy, etc.)
Chickpeas
Chicory
Cowpeas
Lima beans
Spinach
String beans
Turnip greens
Wheat

IRON

There are two types of iron, heme and non-heme. Heme iron, the kind found in animal products, is the easiest for the body to absorb. While there are many vegetables high in iron, they are all non-heme, which the body does not fully absorb. You can enhance your body's ability to absorb the non-heme iron found in legumes and iron-fortified cereals by combining them with meat or foods containing vitamin C. Here are some of the richest sources of iron.

Clams
Cream of wheat

Dry cereal (iron-enriched)
Mussels
Oysters
Poultry
Pumpkin seeds
Red meat
Soybeans
Tofu

MANGANESE

Virtually all whole grains, nuts, and seeds contain manganese. Other top choices of this mineral include these.

Halibut
Pumpkin seeds
Quinoa
Rice bran
Spinach
Sunflower seeds
Tofu
Wheat germ

NIACIN

Any type of poultry and many varieties of fish are good sources of niacin. These are among the best.

Capon
Chicken breast
Halibut
Quail
Rainbow trout
Squab
Swordfish

Tuna
Turkey breast
Veal loin

OMEGA-3 FATTY ACIDS

Fatty cold-water fish are the best sources of omega-3 fatty acids. Poach, bake, or sauté the fish. Deep-fat frying, in addition to adding unnecessary fat, destroys the fatty acids. Top picks include the following.

Anchovies
Atlantic herring
Atlantic mackerel
Atlantic sardines
Bluefin tuna
Pink salmon
Rainbow trout
Sockeye salmon
Swordfish
Tilefish

POTASSIUM

Any kind of fruit or vegetable offers potassium. Among the best sources are these.

Apricots
Avocado
Baked potatoes
Bananas
Beet greens
Clams
Orange juice
Prune juice

Raisins
Yams

PHYTONUTRIENTS

Plant foods contain an abundance of these special nutrients, many of which possess special healing powers. Classes of phytonutrients found in this book and their major food sources include the following.

Ellagic acid
Apples
Berries
Grapes
Green tea

Indoles
Broccoli
Brussels sprouts
Cabbage
Cauliflower
Kale

Isoflavones
Everything soy

Lignans
Flaxseed
Walnuts

Limonoids
Lemons
Limes
Peels of these citrus fruits

Lycopene
    Red grapefruit
    Tomatoes

Phenols
    Blueberries
    Broccoli
    Cabbage
    Tomatoes
    Whole grains

VITAMIN A

Beef liver is the richest source of vitamin A (one serving contains 901% of the DV), but its high cholesterol content is off the charts as well. If you don't have a cholesterol problem, an occasional indulgence is okay. These are better choices.

    Beet greens
    Butternut squash
    Cantaloupe
    Carrots
    Dandelion greens
    Eel
    Lamb
    Mango
    Spinach
    Tuna

VITAMIN B6

Some sources of B6 tend to be high in fat, such as goose liver and sausage. Here are healthier choices.

    Bananas
    Carrot juice

Chicken breast
Chickpeas
Potatoes
Prune juice
Rice bran
Squab
Tuna
Turkey breast

VITAMIN B12

Animal and fish products are loaded with vitamin B12.
The healthiest choices are these.

Alaskan king crab
Atlantic mackerel
Blue crab
Caribou
Clams
Mackerel
Octopus
Rabbit
Sockeye salmon
Tuna

VITAMIN C

Citrus and tropical fruits are the leaders when it comes to
vitamin C. Virtually all of them are chockablock with vitamin C. These are also excellent choices.

Acerola cherries
Bell peppers
Broccoli
Brussels sprouts
Cantaloupe

Currants (black contains the most)
Honeydew melon
Kohlrabi

VITAMIN E

Oils, especially nut oils, are the best sources of vitamin E but you'll want to go for those that are high in monounsaturated fats, which give you a big health boost. Stick with these choices.

Almond oil
Brown rice
Grapeseed oil
Hazelnut oil
Olive oil
Nuts
Peanut oil
Soybean oil
Sunflower oil
Wheat germ

ZINC

Meat and some seafood are the riches source of zinc. But oysters, by far, are the richest choice. In addition to oysters, choose from the following.

Alaskan king crab
Beef round roast
Filet mignon
Lamb shank
Miso
Veal
Wheat germ

APPENDIX B
RESOURCES

NATUROPATHY

A licensed naturopathic physician is a graduate of a four-year, graduate-level naturopathic medical school. Naturopaths learn the same basic sciences that traditional medical doctors do, but their training includes additional coursework in herbal medicine, nutrition, homeopathy, and exercise therapy. Currently, the District of Columbia and 13 states—Alaska, Arizona, California, Connecticut, Hawaii, Kansas, Maine, Montana, New Hampshire, Oregon, Utah, Vermont, and Washington—require that naturopathic physicians pass a state licensing exam.

For a referral to a naturopathic physician in your area, contact:

**The American Association of
Naturopathic Physicians**
3201 New Mexico Avenue, NW
Suite 350
Washington, DC 20016
Toll-free (866) 538–2267; (202) 895–1392
www.naturopathic.org

HOLISTIC MEDICINE

Holistic medicine is practiced by medical doctors, osteopaths, and naturopaths. These physicians emphasize the treatment of the whole person and encourage personal responsibility for health.

For a referral to a licensed holistic practitioner, contact:

The American Holistic Medical Association
12101 Menaul Blvd. NE
Suite C
Albuquerque, NM 87112
(505) 292–7788
www.holisticmedicine.org

The American Holistic Health Association
P.O. Box 17400
Anaheim, CA 92817–7400
(714) 779–6152
www.ahha.org

HERBAL MEDICINE

Herbal medicine is used by many naturopathic physicians and a growing number of conventional doctors. There is no separate certification or licensing process specifically for practitioners of herbal medicine. When choosing a health-care practitioner for advice on herbs, look for someone who is a member of a professional organization, such as the American Herbalists Guild.

For information on herbal medicine and referrals to practitioners in your area, contact:

The American Herbalists Guild
1931 Gaddis Rd.
Canton, GA 30115

(770) 751–6021
www.americanherbalistsguild.com

American Herb Association
P.O. Box 1673
Nevada City, CA 95959
(530) 265–9552
www.ahaherb.com

The American Botanical Council
6200 Manor Rd.
Austin, TX 78723
(800) 373–7105; (512) 926–4900
www.herbalgram.org

Herb Research Foundation
4140 15th Street
Boulder, CO 80304
(303) 449–2265
www.herbs.org

HOMEOPATHY

Homeopathy is practiced by medical doctors, osteopaths, naturopaths, chiropractors, and dentists. Some states also allow chiropractors, family nurse practitioners, acupuncturists, and physician assistants to obtain licensures.

For more information on homeopathy or to locate a homeopath in your area, contact:

The National Center for Homeopathy
801 N. Fairfax Street, Suite 306
Alexandria, VA 22314
(877) 624–0613; (703) 548–7790
www.homeopathic.org

DIET AND NUTRITION

For information on nutrition or to find a qualified nutrition counselor, contact:

The American Association of Nutritional Consultants
400 Oak Hill Dr.
Winona Lake, IN 46590
(888) 828–2262
www.aanc.net

American Dietetic Association
120 South Riverside Plaza, Suite 2000
Chicago, IL 60606–6995
(800) 877–1600
Consumer Nutrition Hotline: (800) 366–1655
www.eatright.org

American Society for Nutritional Sciences
9650 Rockville Pike, Suite 4500
Bethesda, MD 20814–3990
(301) 634–7050
www.asns.org

American Council on Science and Health
1995 Broadway, 2nd Floor
New York, NY 10023–5860
(212) 362–7044
www.acsh.org

Food and Drug Administration
5600 Fishers Lane, HFE 88
Rockville, MD 20857
(888) 463–6332
www.fda.gov

INDEX